The New Carb Cycling for Beginners

Harry Beck

Table of Contents

Introduction 1

Chapter 1: Carb Cycling Basic 2
Understanding the Basics of Carb Cycling 2
How Carb Cycling Differs from Traditional Diets 3
The Science Behind Carb Cycling 4

Chapter 2: The Carb Cycling Diet 5
60-Day Meal Plan 5
High-Carb Days 11
Low-Carb Days 12
Stock-up List 13
Workout Strategies for Success 14
Tracking Your Results 16

Chapter 3: Breakfast Recipes 19
Protein-Packed Pancakes for a Powerful Start 19
Berry Bliss Smoothie Bowl 20
Veggie-packed Frittata Feast 21
Quinoa Power Porridge 22
High-Protein Blueberry Muffins 23
Avocado and Salmon Breakfast Wrap 24
Greek Yogurt Parfait with Nutty Granola 25
Cottage Cheese and Fruit Medley 26
Almond Butter Banana Toast with a Twist 27
Zesty Breakfast Burrito with Lean Turkey 28
Coconut Flour Waffles with Fresh Berries 29

Chapter 4: Snacks and Drinks 30
Nutty Trail Mix Crunch 30
Crunchy Veggie Sticks with Hummus 31
Hard-Boiled Eggs with a Kick 32
Almond and Coconut Energy Bites 33
Spicy Roasted Chickpeas Snack 34
Avocado Salsa with Whole Grain Crackers 35
Cucumber Slices with Tzatziki Dip 36

Guacamole-Stuffed Cherry Tomatoes 37
Greek Yogurt and Berry Smoothie.. 38
Green Tea Infusion for Antioxidant Boost 39
Fresh Fruit Kabobs with Mint Yogurt Dip 39
Iced Herbal Infusion with Citrus Twist.. 40
Berry Blast Protein Shake 41
Minty Matcha Latte 42
Tropical Pineapple Coconut Smoothie 43
Refreshing Cucumber Mint Cooler 44

Chapter 5: Beef, Pork, and Poultry Recipes 45
Grilled Lemon-Herb Chicken Breast 45
Savory Garlic and Rosemary Beef Skewers 46
Mediterranean Turkey Meatballs 47
Citrus-Marinated Grilled Pork Chops 48
Spicy Sriracha Chicken Stir-Fry 49
Lean Beef and Vegetable Stuffed Peppers 50
Tangy Teriyaki Chicken Thighs.. 51
Zesty Lime and Cilantro Turkey Burgers... 52
Slow-Cooked Italian Herb Pulled Pork.. 53
Sesame-Ginger Glazed Chicken Drumsticks... 54
Chipotle Lime Grilled Steak Strips 55

Chapter 6: Fish and Seafood Recipes 56
Lemon-Garlic Grilled Salmon 56
Spicy Shrimp and Zucchini Noodles.. 57
Baked Cod with Herbed Quinoa... 58
Teriyaki Glazed Tuna Steaks 59
Citrus Herb Grilled Sea Bass 60
Garlic Butter Shrimp Skewers... 61
Coconut-Crusted Tilapia Bites 62
Cajun-Style Blackened Catfish 63
Sesame Ginger Marinated Scallops 64
Mediterranean Herb Baked Trout 65
Lime Cilantro Grilled Swordfish.. 66

Chapter 7: Pasta and Soups 67
Whole Wheat Penne with Roasted Vegetables.. 67
Turmeric Infused Lentil Soup.. 68
Zucchini Noodles with Turkey Bolognese 69

Roasted Red Pepper and Tomato Soup 70
Spinach and Mushroom Quinoa Risotto 71
Thai Coconut Curry Shrimp Soup 72
Spaghetti Squash Carbonara 73
Spicy Cauliflower and Chickpea Soup 74
Eggplant and Tomato Linguine 75
Lemon Dill Chicken and Orzo Soup 76

Chapter 8: Vegan and Vegeratian **77**
Quinoa and Black Bean Stuffed Bell Peppers 77
Lentil and Vegetable Curry 78
Zucchini Noodles with Vegan Pesto 79
Chickpea and Spinach Coconut Curry 80
Roasted Vegetable and Hummus Wrap 81
Sweet Potato and Black Bean Enchiladas 82
Mediterranean Chickpea Salad 83
Portobello Mushroom and Quinoa Burgers 84
Vegan Thai Green Curry with Tofu 85
Spinach and Mushroom Quinoa Risotto 86
Vegan Chickpea and Sweet Potato Chili 87

Chapter 9: Desserts **88**
Dark Chocolate Avocado Mousse 88
Coconut Flour Banana Bread 89
Protein-Packed Peanut Butter Cookies 90
Lemon Blueberry Protein Muffins 91
Almond Flour Chocolate Chip Blondies 92
Pumpkin Spice Energy Bites 93
Apple Cinnamon Quinoa Bake 94
Avocado Chocolate Pudding Cups 95
Vanilla Protein Ice Cream 96
Mango Coconut Rice Pudding 97

Chapter 10: Dining Out and Social Events **98**

Chapter 11: Approach for Long-Term Success **99**

2. Bonus Chapters: **100**
1. Creating Balanced and Nutrient-Dense Meals 100
2. Advanced Strategies: Graduating to Advanced Carb Cycling 103

Conclusion **105**

Introduction

Embark on a transformative journey towards optimal health and fitness with "The New Carb Cycling for Beginners," a groundbreaking guide meticulously designed for those seeking a revolutionary approach to nutrition. In a world saturated with fad diets and conflicting information, this comprehensive resource stands out as a beacon of clarity, offering a fresh perspective on how controlled carbohydrate consumption can reshape your body and energize your life.

As the fitness landscape evolves, so does our understanding of nutrition, and carb cycling emerges as a dynamic strategy at the forefront of this paradigm shift. This book serves as a gateway for beginners, introducing them to a nuanced and effective method that goes beyond the limitations of traditional dieting norms.

To further enhance the reader's experience, we've included a chapter titled "60-Day Meal Plan." This provides a tangible roadmap for applying carb cycling principles in daily life, offering sample meal plans tailored for various goals. From breakfast recipes that kickstart your day to delicious desserts that align with your nutritional targets, this chapter makes the transition to carb cycling seamless and delicious.

In conclusion, "The New Carb Cycling for Beginners" isn't just a book; it's a transformative guide that empowers you to take charge of your health and fitness. With a revolutionary approach backed by science, practical guidance, and sustainable practices, this book invites you to embrace a new way of thinking about nutrition—one that will pave the way for lasting success on your fitness journey. So, are you ready to unlock the transformative potential of carb cycling and craft a future that is both lighter and happier? The journey begins now; turn the page and step into a new chapter of your life.

Chapter 1:
Carb Cycling Basic

Understanding the Basics of Carb Cycling

Embark on a transformative journey into the realm of nutrition with our in-depth exploration of the fundamentals of carb cycling. This comprehensive guide aims to demystify the intricacies of carb cycling, offering a beacon of clarity for individuals at all stages of their fitness journey. Whether you're a newcomer seeking to decipher the buzz surrounding carb cycling or a seasoned enthusiast looking to deepen your understanding, this chapter serves as your compass, guiding you through the core principles of this dynamic dietary strategy.

At its essence, carb cycling involves strategically adjusting your carbohydrate intake throughout the week, aiming to optimize energy levels, enhance fat loss, and support muscle growth. This approach acknowledges that one size does not fit all when it comes to nutrition, recognizing the dynamic nature of our bodies and the varying demands placed upon them.

Delve into the heart of carb cycling by exploring its core concepts. Learn how to distinguish high-carb days from low-carb days and understand the impact of these fluctuations on your metabolism. Uncover the science behind carb cycling, shedding light on how it influences key hormones and metabolic pathways. As we unravel the mysteries, you'll gain valuable insights into why carb cycling stands apart from traditional diets, offering a flexible and sustainable approach to achieving your health and fitness goals.

The journey begins with an assessment of your fitness level and goals. This crucial step lays the foundation for tailoring a carb cycling plan that aligns with your unique needs. Whether your aim is to shed excess body fat, build lean muscle, or optimize athletic performance, understanding how to assess and set realistic goals is the cornerstone of a successful carb cycling journey.

Once armed with this foundational knowledge, we navigate the practical aspects of carb cycling, from creating balanced and nutrient-dense meals to seamlessly integrating this approach into your daily life. Explore a diverse array of meal plans designed for various goals, providing you with a roadmap for success. From breakfast recipes that kickstart your metabolism to delicious desserts that satisfy your sweet tooth without compromising your progress, each meal is crafted to strike the perfect balance of macronutrients to support your objectives.

As you dive into the world of carb cycling, workout strategies tailored for success become paramount. Discover how to synchronize your exercise routine with your carb cycling plan, maximizing the benefits of both. Whether you're engaging in high-intensity interval training (HIIT) or prefer a more moderate approach, adapting your workouts to complement your nutritional strategy is key to unlocking the full potential of carb cycling.

However, every journey encounters challenges, and carb cycling is no exception. This chapter equips you with the tools to troubleshoot issues, overcome plateaus, and adjust your approach for long-term success. Common challenges are addressed with practical solutions, ensuring that you can navigate the inevitable bumps in the road on your path to optimal health and fitness.

Going beyond the basics, we delve into advanced strategies, exploring how to graduate to an advanced level of carb cycling. Understand the nuances of an advanced approach, allowing you to fine-tune your carb cycling plan for even more targeted results. The journey doesn't end with mastery; it evolves as you continue your pursuit of optimal health and fitness.

In conclusion, "Understanding the Basics of Carb Cycling" is your comprehensive roadmap to a nuanced and effective nutritional strategy. It empowers you with the knowledge to customize your approach, ensuring that carb cycling seamlessly integrates into your lifestyle, unlocking the transformative potential for a healthier, more vibrant you.

How Carb Cycling Differs from Traditional Diets

Dive into the dynamic world of nutrition and discover how carb cycling stands as a beacon of innovation in contrast to traditional diet approaches. Unlike one-size-fits-all regimens, carb cycling is a personalized strategy that acknowledges the varying needs of our bodies. While conventional diets often impose a rigid structure, carb cycling introduces flexibility by strategically alternating between higher and lower carbohydrate days.

The key distinction lies in recognizing that carbohydrates are not the enemy; rather, they are a crucial component of a balanced diet. Carb cycling optimizes the timing and quantity of carbohydrate intake, leveraging their energy-boosting properties without leading to excess storage. This nuanced approach taps into the science of metabolism, acknowledging that our bodies respond differently to varying macronutrient ratios.

Traditional diets often enforce a constant caloric restriction, potentially leading to metabolic adaptation and plateaus in weight loss. In contrast, carb cycling employs a cyclical approach, challenging the body to adapt and optimize its metabolic efficiency. On high-carb days, energy levels soar, promoting effective workouts and muscle building. Conversely, low-carb days encourage the body to tap into stored fat for fuel, facilitating fat loss while maintaining muscle mass.

Moreover, carb cycling recognizes the importance of individual goals and activity levels. Tailoring carbohydrate intake to align with specific fitness objectives ensures a sustainable approach that accommodates both weight loss and muscle gain aspirations. This adaptability sets carb cycling apart as a lifestyle-oriented strategy, fostering a healthy relationship with food rather than imposing strict rules.

In essence, the beauty of carb cycling lies in its ability to harmonize nutritional principles with individual needs. It offers a refreshing departure from the rigidity of traditional diets, providing a flexible and sustainable approach to achieving health and fitness goals. As we delve into the intricacies of carb cycling, a new paradigm emerges—one that invites you to embrace the power of customization and balance in your nutritional journey.

The Science Behind Carb Cycling

Embark on a journey into the intricate science that underlies the transformative power of carb cycling. At its core, carb cycling strategically manipulates your carbohydrate intake, recognizing the dynamic nature of our bodies' responses to varying macronutrient ratios. Delve into the impact on insulin levels, hormonal regulation, and metabolic pathways as you explore the interplay between high and low-carb days.

High-carb days are orchestrated to capitalize on increased insulin sensitivity, fostering an environment conducive to muscle growth and optimal workout performance. On these days, elevated energy levels fuel rigorous training sessions, promoting muscle protein synthesis. Conversely, low-carb days prompt the body to tap into stored fat for fuel, facilitating fat loss without compromising muscle mass.

Understanding the intricacies of carb cycling empowers you to synchronize nutrition with your fitness goals. The cyclical nature challenges the body to adapt, preventing metabolic stagnation often encountered with continuous caloric restriction. This chapter provides a roadmap to harness the benefits of increased metabolic flexibility, allowing you to efficiently switch between utilizing carbohydrates and fats for energy.

As you navigate through the scientific principles, you'll gain a profound comprehension of how carb cycling becomes a strategic ally in achieving a leaner, more resilient physique. The tailored manipulation of carbohydrate intake emerges not as a one-size-fits-all solution but as a nuanced strategy that harmonizes with your body's unique requirements, paving the way for sustained health and fitness success.

Chapter 2:
The Carb Cycling Diet

60-Day Meal Plan

Day	Breakfast	Lunch	Dinner	Snack
1	Protein-Packed Pancakes for a Powerful Start	Grilled Lemon-Herb Chicken Breast	Lemon-Garlic Grilled Salmon	Nutty Trail Mix Crunch
2	Berry Bliss Smoothie Bowl	Savory Garlic and Rosemary Beef Skewers	Spicy Shrimp and Zucchini Noodles	Crunchy Veggie Sticks with Hummus
3	Veggie-packed Frittata Feast	Quinoa and Black Bean Stuffed Bell Peppers	Vegan Thai Green Curry with Tofu	Hard-Boiled Eggs with a Kick
4	Quinoa Power Porridge	Citrus-Marinated Grilled Pork Chops	Teriyaki Glazed Tuna Steaks	Almond and Coconut Energy Bites
5	High-Protein Blueberry Muffins	Spicy Sriracha Chicken Stir-Fry	Citrus Herb Grilled Sea Bass	Spicy Roasted Chickpeas Snack
6	Avocado and Salmon Breakfast Wrap	Lean Beef and Vegetable Stuffed Peppers	Garlic Butter Shrimp Skewers	Avocado Salsa with Whole Grain Crackers
7	Greek Yogurt Parfait with Nutty Granola	Tangy Teriyaki Chicken Thighs	Coconut-Crusted Tilapia Bites	Cucumber Slices with Tzatziki Dip
8	Cottage Cheese and Fruit Medley	Zesty Lime and Cilantro Turkey Burgers	Cajun-Style Blackened Catfish	Guacamole-Stuffed Cherry Tomatoes

9	Almond Butter Banana Toast with a Twist	Slow-Cooked Italian Herb Pulled Pork	Sesame Ginger Marinated Scallops	Greek Yogurt and Berry Smoothie	
10	Zesty Breakfast Burrito with Lean Turkey	Sesame-Ginger Glazed Chicken Drumsticks	Mediterranean Herb Baked Trout	Green Tea Infusion for Antioxidant Boost	
11	Coconut Flour Waffles with Fresh Berries	Chipotle Lime Grilled Steak Strips	Lime Cilantro Grilled Swordfish	Fresh Fruit Kabobs with Mint Yogurt Dip	
12	Protein-Packed Pancakes for a Powerful Start	Whole Wheat Penne with Roasted Vegetables	Roasted Vegetable and Hummus Wrap	Iced Herbal Infusion with Citrus Twist	
13	Berry Bliss Smoothie Bowl	Turmeric Infused Lentil Soup	Sweet Potato and Black Bean Enchiladas	Berry Blast Protein Shake	
14	Veggie-packed Frittata Feast	Zucchini Noodles with Turkey Bolognese	Mediterranean Chickpea Salad	Minty Matcha Latte	
15	Quinoa Power Porridge	Roasted Red Pepper and Tomato Soup	Cajun-Style Blackened Catfish	Tropical Pineapple Coconut Smoothie	
16	High-Protein Blueberry Muffins	Spinach and Mushroom Quinoa Risotto	Sesame Ginger Marinated Scallops	Refreshing Cucumber Mint Cooler	
17	Avocado and Salmon Breakfast Wrap	Thai Coconut Curry Shrimp Soup	Mediterranean Herb Baked Trout	Nutty Trail Mix Crunch	
18	Greek Yogurt Parfait with Nutty Granola	Spaghetti Squash Carbonara	Lime Cilantro Grilled Swordfish	Crunchy Veggie Sticks with Hummus	

19	Cottage Cheese and Fruit Medley	Spicy Cauliflower and Chickpea Soup	Roasted Vegetable and Hummus Wrap	Hard-Boiled Eggs with a Kick	
20	Almond Butter Banana Toast with a Twist	Eggplant and Tomato Linguine	Vegan Chickpea and Sweet Potato Chili	Almond and Coconut Energy Bites	
21	Zesty Breakfast Burrito with Lean Turkey	Lemon Dill Chicken and Orzo Soup	Spicy Shrimp and Zucchini Noodles	Spicy Roasted Chickpeas Snack	
22	Coconut Flour Waffles with Fresh Berries	Mediterranean Turkey Meatballs	Baked Cod with Herbed Quinoa	Avocado Salsa with Whole Grain Crackers	
23	Protein-Packed Pancakes for a Powerful Start	Whole Wheat Penne with Roasted Vegetables	Grilled Lemon-Herb Chicken Breast	Cucumber Slices with Tzatziki Dip	
24	Berry Bliss Smoothie Bowl	Turmeric Infused Lentil Soup	Savory Garlic and Rosemary Beef Skewers	Guacamole-Stuffed Cherry Tomatoes	
25	Veggie-packed Frittata Feast	Lentil and Vegetable Curry	Teriyaki Glazed Tuna Steaks	Greek Yogurt and Berry Smoothie	
26	Quinoa Power Porridge	Zucchini Noodles with Vegan Pesto	Citrus Herb Grilled Sea Bass	Green Tea Infusion for Antioxidant Boost	
27	High-Protein Blueberry Muffins	Chickpea and Spinach Coconut Curry	Garlic Butter Shrimp Skewers	Fresh Fruit Kabobs with Mint Yogurt Dip	
28	Avocado and Salmon Breakfast Wrap	Roasted Vegetable and Hummus Wrap	Citrus-Marinated Grilled Pork Chops	Iced Herbal Infusion with Citrus Twist	

29	Greek Yogurt Parfait with Nutty Granola	Sweet Potato and Black Bean Enchiladas	Spicy Sriracha Chicken Stir-Fry	Berry Blast Protein Shake	
30	Cottage Cheese and Fruit Medley	Mediterranean Chickpea Salad	Lean Beef and Vegetable Stuffed Peppers	Minty Matcha Latte	
31	Almond Butter Banana Toast with a Twist	Portobello Mushroom and Quinoa Burgers	Tangy Teriyaki Chicken Thighs	Tropical Pineapple Coconut Smoothie	
32	Zesty Breakfast Burrito with Lean Turkey	Vegan Thai Green Curry with Tofu	Zesty Lime and Cilantro Turkey Burgers	Refreshing Cucumber Mint Cooler	
33	Coconut Flour Waffles with Fresh Berries	Spinach and Mushroom Quinoa Risotto	Slow-Cooked Italian Herb Pulled Pork	Nutty Trail Mix Crunch	
34	Protein-Packed Pancakes for a Powerful Start	Vegan Chickpea and Sweet Potato Chili	Lemon-Garlic Grilled Salmon	Crunchy Veggie Sticks with Hummus	
35	Berry Bliss Smoothie Bowl	Garlic Butter Shrimp Skewers	Spicy Shrimp and Zucchini Noodles	Hard-Boiled Eggs with a Kick	
36	Veggie-packed Frittata Feast	Zucchini Noodles with Turkey Bolognese	Mediterranean Chickpea Salad	Almond and Coconut Energy Bites	
37	Quinoa Power Porridge	Roasted Red Pepper and Tomato Soup	Cajun-Style Blackened Catfish	Spicy Roasted Chickpeas Snack	
38	High-Protein Blueberry Muffins	Spinach and Mushroom Quinoa Risotto	Sesame Ginger Marinated Scallops	Avocado Salsa with Whole Grain Crackers	

39	Avocado and Salmon Breakfast Wrap	Thai Coconut Curry Shrimp Soup	Mediterranean Herb Baked Trout	Cucumber Slices with Tzatziki Dip	
40	Greek Yogurt Parfait with Nutty Granola	Spaghetti Squash Carbonara	Lime Cilantro Grilled Swordfish	Guacamole-Stuffed Cherry Tomatoes	
41	Cottage Cheese and Fruit Medley	Spicy Cauliflower and Chickpea Soup	Roasted Vegetable and Hummus Wrap	Greek Yogurt and Berry Smoothie	
42	Almond Butter Banana Toast with a Twist	Eggplant and Tomato Linguine	Vegan Chickpea and Sweet Potato Chili	Green Tea Infusion for Antioxidant Boost	
43	Zesty Breakfast Burrito with Lean Turkey	Turmeric Infused Lentil Soup	Savory Garlic and Rosemary Beef Skewers	Fresh Fruit Kabobs with Mint Yogurt Dip	
44	Coconut Flour Waffles with Fresh Berries	Lentil and Vegetable Curry	Teriyaki Glazed Tuna Steaks	Iced Herbal Infusion with Citrus Twist	
45	Protein-Packed Pancakes for a Powerful Start	Zucchini Noodles with Vegan Pesto	Citrus Herb Grilled Sea Bass	Berry Blast Protein Shake	
46	Berry Bliss Smoothie Bowl	Chickpea and Spinach Coconut Curry	Garlic Butter Shrimp Skewers	Minty Matcha Latte	
47	Veggie-packed Frittata Feast	Roasted Vegetable and Hummus Wrap	Citrus-Marinated Grilled Pork Chops	Tropical Pineapple Coconut Smoothie	
48	Quinoa Power Porridge	Citrus-Marinated Grilled Pork Chops	Teriyaki Glazed Tuna Steaks	Refreshing Cucumber Mint Cooler	

49	High-Protein Blueberry Muffins	Spicy Sriracha Chicken Stir-Fry	Citrus Herb Grilled Sea Bass	Nutty Trail Mix Crunch	
50	Avocado and Salmon Breakfast Wrap	Lean Beef and Vegetable Stuffed Peppers	Garlic Butter Shrimp Skewers	Crunchy Veggie Sticks with Hummus	
51	Greek Yogurt Parfait with Nutty Granola	Tangy Teriyaki Chicken Thighs	Coconut-Crusted Tilapia Bites	Hard-Boiled Eggs with a Kick	
52	Cottage Cheese and Fruit Medley	Zesty Lime and Cilantro Turkey Burgers	Cajun-Style Blackened Catfish	Almond and Coconut Energy Bites	
53	Almond Butter Banana Toast with a Twist	Slow-Cooked Italian Herb Pulled Pork	Sesame Ginger Marinated Scallops	Spicy Roasted Chickpeas Snack	
54	Zesty Breakfast Burrito with Lean Turkey	Sesame-Ginger Glazed Chicken Drumsticks	Mediterranean Herb Baked Trout	Avocado Salsa with Whole Grain Crackers	
55	Coconut Flour Waffles with Fresh Berries	Chipotle Lime Grilled Steak Strips	Lime Cilantro Grilled Swordfish	Cucumber Slices with Tzatziki Dip	
56	Protein-Packed Pancakes for a Powerful Start	Thai Coconut Curry Shrimp Soup	Mediterranean Herb Baked Trout	Guacamole-Stuffed Cherry Tomatoes	
57	Berry Bliss Smoothie Bowl	Spaghetti Squash Carbonara	Lime Cilantro Grilled Swordfish	Greek Yogurt and Berry Smoothie	
58	Veggie-packed Frittata Feast	Spicy Cauliflower and Chickpea Soup	Roasted Vegetable and Hummus Wrap	Green Tea Infusion for Antioxidant Boost	
59	Quinoa Power Porridge	Lean Beef and Vegetable	Garlic Butter Shrimp Skewers	Fresh Fruit Kabobs with	

		Stuffed Peppers		Mint Yogurt Dip	
60	High-Protein Blueberry Muffins	Tangy Teriyaki Chicken Thighs	Coconut-Crusted Tilapia Bites	Iced Herbal Infusion with Citrus Twist	

High-Carb Days

In the realm of the carb cycling diet, there exists a strategic and invigorating phase that plays a pivotal role in optimizing energy levels and fueling workouts—let's refer to it as the "Energetic Phase." During this period, the emphasis is on strategically incorporating a higher intake of carbohydrates into your nutrition plan. The rationale behind this lies in the body's response to increased carbohydrate consumption, leading to elevated glycogen levels. Glycogen, stored in the muscles and liver, serves as a primary energy source during intense physical activities.

The Energetic Phase is strategically timed to coincide with your more demanding workout routines or physically challenging days. By capitalizing on increased carbohydrate availability, your body is better equipped to meet the energy demands of these activities, ultimately enhancing your overall performance. This phase aligns with the fundamental principle of carb cycling, which advocates for a cyclical approach to carbohydrate intake based on the fluctuations in your energy requirements.

During the Energetic Phase, your carbohydrate sources become diverse and nutrient-rich, emphasizing complex carbohydrates that release energy gradually. This includes whole grains, legumes, and a variety of colorful vegetables. This nuanced selection aims not only to replenish glycogen stores efficiently but also to provide a spectrum of essential vitamins, minerals, and fiber crucial for overall well-being.

It's essential to view the Energetic Phase not as a departure from a balanced diet but as a purposeful adjustment to support your body's varying needs throughout the carb cycling cycle. This approach fosters metabolic flexibility, encouraging your body to efficiently switch between utilizing carbohydrates and fat for fuel, a key aspect of the carb cycling methodology.

In addition to its physiological benefits, the Energetic Phase contributes to a positive psychological aspect of the carb cycling journey. Enjoying a higher carbohydrate intake on specific days not only adds variety to your diet but also provides a welcomed mental break, preventing the monotony that can accompany rigid nutrition plans.

As with any aspect of the carb cycling diet, individualization is key. The Energetic Phase should be tailored to your unique preferences, energy demands, and fitness goals. Monitoring your body's response and adjusting the quantity and timing of carbohydrates accordingly ensures that you reap the maximum benefits of this phase.

In conclusion, the Energetic Phase embodies a purposeful and dynamic approach to carbohydrate intake within the carb cycling framework. By strategically incorporating higher carbohydrate days, you harness the power of nutrition to optimize your performance, support metabolic flexibility, and introduce a welcomed variety to your dietary routine—all contributing factors to a successful and sustainable carb cycling journey.

Low-Carb Days

In the domain of carb cycling, there exists a purposeful and transformative phase known as the "Energetic Phase," where strategic adjustments to carbohydrate intake become the focal point. However, complementing this dynamic cycle is an equally crucial and contrasting phase—let's call it the "Balanced Resilience Phase." During this period, the emphasis shifts towards a mindful reduction in carbohydrate intake, creating a metabolic environment that encourages the body to tap into alternative energy sources, namely stored fats.

The Balanced Resilience Phase strategically aligns with days that may involve less strenuous physical activity or serve as rest and recovery periods. By deliberately moderating carbohydrate consumption during these intervals, the body is prompted to enter a state of ketosis, where it begins to utilize stored fat as a primary fuel source. This metabolic shift not only contributes to the mobilization of fat stores but also supports a more stable blood sugar level, promoting sustained energy throughout the day.

This phase embodies a nuanced selection of nutrient-dense foods, emphasizing high-quality proteins, healthy fats, and a spectrum of non-starchy vegetables. By diversifying nutrient sources, the Balanced Resilience Phase aims to provide essential vitamins, minerals, and antioxidants crucial for overall well-being.

Importantly, viewing this phase as an intentional adjustment rather than a departure from a balanced diet is key. It aligns with the fundamental principles of carb cycling, promoting adaptability and metabolic flexibility. By periodically restricting carbohydrate intake, you encourage your body to become adept at efficiently utilizing both carbohydrates and fats for energy, a cornerstone of the carb cycling methodology.

Beyond its physiological benefits, the Balanced Resilience Phase introduces a mental resilience aspect to the carb cycling journey. Embracing lower carbohydrate days offers an opportunity for heightened mindfulness around food choices and cultivates a conscious awareness of the body's response to various nutritional inputs. This mindfulness extends beyond the phase itself, influencing long-term dietary habits and promoting a healthier relationship with food.

As with any aspect of the carb cycling diet, individualization remains paramount. Tailoring the Balanced Resilience Phase to your unique preferences, energy demands, and fitness goals ensures a personalized approach that aligns seamlessly with your overall carb cycling journey. Monitoring your body's response and adjusting dietary parameters accordingly enhances the efficacy of this phase, allowing you to reap the maximum benefits of this intentional nutritional strategy.

In conclusion, the Balanced Resilience Phase encapsulates a purposeful reduction in carbohydrate intake within the carb cycling framework. By strategically implementing lower carbohydrate days, you empower your body to optimize fat metabolism, stabilize energy levels, and foster a resilient and mindful approach to nutrition—a multifaceted strategy contributing to the success and sustainability of your carb cycling journey.

Stock-up List

The concept of a "Stock-up List" emerges as a strategic and empowering tool, shaping your journey towards optimal health and fitness. This curated list is not just a mere compilation of groceries; it is a thoughtful selection of nutritionally dense and versatile items designed to support you through both the Energetic and Balanced Resilience Phases of the carb cycling cycle.

At the heart of the Stock-up List is a focus on high-quality proteins, essential for muscle repair and maintenance. Options such as lean meats, poultry, fish, and plant-based protein sources ensure a diverse array of amino acids to support your body's needs during both phases. Complementing this protein foundation are healthy fats from sources like avocados, nuts, and olive oil, providing sustained energy and promoting satiety.

The inclusion of a variety of non-starchy vegetables is a key feature, aligning with the principles of both phases. These colorful gems not only contribute essential vitamins, minerals, and antioxidants but also offer a low-calorie, high-fiber profile, supporting digestive health and providing a sense of fullness.

Whole grains find their place on the Stock-up List, supplying complex carbohydrates for the Energetic Phase. These grains, such as quinoa, brown rice, and oats, release energy gradually, ensuring a sustained fuel source for your more demanding workout days. Conversely, the list acknowledges the importance of reducing carbohydrate intake on low carb days, encouraging the consumption of nutrient-dense alternatives like cauliflower rice and spiralized vegetables.

The Stock-up List is a dynamic guide, accommodating dietary preferences and ensuring flexibility. It opens the door to exploring a spectrum of nutrient-rich foods, fostering a holistic approach to nutrition. From dairy or dairy alternatives for calcium and vitamin D to a selection of herbs and spices for flavor without added calories, this list empowers you to create well-balanced and enjoyable meals throughout your carb cycling journey.

Importantly, the Stock-up List is not a rigid prescription but a tool for customization. It encourages mindfulness around food choices, empowering you to make informed decisions that align with your individual tastes and nutritional requirements. By keeping your pantry and refrigerator stocked with these versatile and nutritious options, you set yourself up for success, ensuring that you have the building blocks to create delicious, balanced meals in line with the principles of carb cycling.

In conclusion, the Stock-up List transcends the conventional notion of a grocery list. It is a dynamic and purposeful collection of foods strategically chosen to support the intricacies of the carb cycling diet. By embracing the variety and nutritional richness it offers, you equip yourself with the essentials to navigate the diverse phases of carb cycling, creating a foundation for sustained health, fitness, and enjoyment along the way.

Workout Strategies for Success

Effective workout strategies stand as the linchpin to amplify your success and propel you toward your fitness goals. This chapter, aptly titled "Workout Strategies for Success," serves as your comprehensive guide to navigating the symbiotic relationship between exercise and carb cycling, unlocking the full potential of your fitness journey.

Understanding that exercise is not a one-size-fits-all endeavor, this chapter delves into tailoring your workout routines to align seamlessly with the dynamic principles of carb cycling. Whether you're embracing a high-energy, high-carb day or adopting a more resilient, low-carb approach, the goal is to synchronize your nutritional intake with the varying demands of your exercise regimen.

For the energetic phases, where carbohydrate availability is at its peak, the focus shifts to high-intensity workouts that capitalize on the body's enhanced capacity to utilize carbohydrates as a primary fuel source. This might involve engaging in vigorous cardio sessions, weightlifting, or interval training to maximize glycogen utilization and optimize energy levels. The chapter provides a curated selection of workout routines and tips tailored specifically for these high-energy days, ensuring that you make the most of your nutritional resources.

Conversely, during the more resilient phases with reduced carbohydrate intake, the emphasis shifts to workouts that tap into alternative energy sources, such as stored fats. Incorporating lower-intensity cardio, endurance activities, or even incorporating elements of resistance training, these strategies optimize fat metabolism while still providing effective and sustainable exercise options. The chapter offers a diverse array of low-carb workout suggestions, empowering you to maintain momentum and endurance even on days with a lower carbohydrate focus.

Central to the success of these workout strategies is the concept of metabolic flexibility—the body's ability to efficiently switch between utilizing carbohydrates and fats for fuel. By aligning your exercise routines with the principles of carb cycling, you encourage this adaptive flexibility, promoting overall metabolic efficiency and supporting your fitness goals.

Beyond the specific exercises, the chapter delves into the importance of pre- and post-workout nutrition, emphasizing the role of carbohydrates, proteins, and fats in optimizing performance and facilitating recovery. Practical tips on hydration, supplementation, and timing provide actionable insights to enhance the effectiveness of your workouts within the carb cycling framework.

This chapter isn't just about prescribing workouts; it's about empowering you to create a personalized and sustainable fitness routine that complements the nuances of the carb cycling diet. By embracing the synergistic relationship between nutrition and exercise, you'll not only maximize the benefits of carb cycling but also cultivate a holistic approach to health and fitness that lasts. So, lace up those sneakers, grab your water bottle, and let the workout strategies in this chapter propel you toward success on your carb cycling journey.

Examples of workouts:

1. High Carb Days:

Intense Cardio Workouts:

- High-intensity interval training (HIIT)
- Running or sprinting sessions
- Cycling at a fast pace

Strength Training:

- Weightlifting with moderate to heavy weights
- Circuit training incorporating resistance exercises
- Full-body workout routines

Post-Workout Nutrition:

- Protein and carbohydrate-rich shake or smoothie
- Balanced meal with lean protein, whole grains, and vegetables

2. Low Carb Days:

Moderate-Intensity Cardio:

- Brisk walking or hiking
- Cycling at a steady pace

- Swimming or water aerobics

Endurance Activities:

- Long-distance running or jogging
- Extended cycling or spinning sessions
- Low-impact aerobic workouts

Resistance Training:

- Bodyweight exercises (push-ups, squats, lunges)
- Yoga or Pilates
- Lighter weight, higher rep weightlifting

Post-Workout Nutrition:

- Protein-rich snack or meal
- Emphasis on healthy fats and lean proteins
- Hydration with water or electrolyte-rich beverages

3. Overall Considerations:

Timing of Workouts:

- Consider aligning more demanding workouts with high carb days.
- Plan lower intensity or recovery workouts on low carb days.

Hydration:

- Maintain consistent hydration throughout all phases.
- Consider electrolyte-rich beverages for intense workouts.

Pre-Workout Nutrition:

- Include a balanced mix of carbohydrates and proteins before workouts.
- Tailor pre-workout nutrition based on the upcoming phase.

Adaptation and Flexibility:

- Pay attention to how your body responds and adjust accordingly.
- Modify workout intensity and duration based on energy levels.

Tracking Your Results

Tracking your results is not just a practice; it's a powerful tool that empowers you to understand the nuances of how your body responds to different phases and adjustments in your nutrition and exercise routine. This chapter, aptly titled "Tracking Your Results," serves as your compass in this transformative journey, providing guidance on monitoring key metrics and making informed decisions for continuous progress.

One of the fundamental aspects of result tracking is keeping a comprehensive food diary. By diligently recording your daily meals, including the types and quantities of carbohydrates consumed, you gain valuable insights into the relationship between your nutrition choices and energy levels, mood, and overall well-being. Modern technology makes this process more accessible than ever, with numerous apps allowing you to log meals effortlessly and analyze nutritional content.

Beyond just noting down what you eat, it's essential to track how your body feels and performs. This involves keeping a workout journal where you record the details of each exercise session, noting the intensity, duration, and any notable changes in strength or endurance. Tracking your energy levels throughout the day provides additional context, helping you identify patterns and correlations between nutrition, workouts, and overall vitality.

Measuring physical progress is a tangible way to validate the effectiveness of your carb cycling journey. Utilize tools such as body measurements, photographs, and body composition assessments to track changes in muscle mass and fat percentage. While the scale can be a useful metric, it's crucial not to rely solely on weight as fluctuations can occur due to various factors, including water retention and muscle gain.

Incorporating biofeedback markers into your tracking routine provides a holistic view of your body's responses. Monitoring sleep quality, stress levels, and mood fluctuations offers valuable insights into how external factors impact your overall well-being and, subsequently, your fitness journey. There are wearable devices and apps designed to assist in tracking these biofeedback markers, creating a more comprehensive picture of your health.

As you embark on carb cycling, consider setting specific, measurable, achievable, relevant, and time-bound (SMART) goals. Whether it's achieving a certain body fat percentage, improving your mile time, or mastering a new fitness skill, clearly defined goals serve as benchmarks for success and motivation. Regularly revisit and adjust these goals based on your evolving fitness level and aspirations.

To illustrate, let's say your initial goal is to reduce body fat. You might track this by taking monthly body measurements, capturing progress photos, and using body fat calipers for a more precise assessment. Pairing this with a goal to increase energy levels during workouts allows you to correlate dietary changes with performance improvements.

In conclusion, "Tracking Your Results" is not just about numbers; it's about gaining a deep understanding of your body's responses to the intricacies of carb cycling. Embrace the wealth of tools and technologies available to you, tailor them to your preferences, and let the insights gleaned guide your decisions for a more informed and successful carb cycling journey.

Sample table to track your results:

Date	Consumed Foods	Physical Activity	Weight	Notes

Chapter 3: Breakfast Recipes

Protein-Packed Pancakes for a Powerful Start

Preparation time: 10 minutes

Cooking time: 10 minutes

Servings: 2

Ingredients:

- 1 cup whole wheat flour
- 1 scoop protein powder
- 1 tablespoon honey
- 1 teaspoon baking powder
- 1 cup almond milk
- 1 egg
- 1 teaspoon vanilla extract
- Cooking spray

Instructions:

1. In a bowl, whisk together the flour, protein powder, baking powder, almond milk, egg, honey, and vanilla extract until well combined.
2. Heat a griddle or non-stick pan over medium heat and coat with cooking spray.
3. Pour 1/4 cup of batter onto the griddle for each pancake.
4. Cook until bubbles form on the surface, then flip and cook until golden brown.
5. Serve with your favorite berries and a drizzle of honey.

Nutritional Information (per serving): Calories: 350kcal; Fat: 10g; Carbs: 45g; Protein: 20g

Berry Bliss Smoothie Bowl

Preparation time: 5 minutes

Servings: 2

Ingredients:

- 1 cup mixed berries (strawberries, blueberries, raspberries)
- 1 frozen banana
- 1/2 cup Greek yogurt
- 1/2 cup almond milk
- 1 tablespoon chia seeds
- 1 tablespoon honey
- Granola and sliced almonds for topping

Instructions:

1. In a blender, combine the mixed berries, frozen banana, Greek yogurt, almond milk, chia seeds, and honey.
2. Blend until smooth and creamy.
3. Pour the smoothie into bowls and top with granola and sliced almonds.
4. Enjoy this refreshing and nutritious smoothie bowl.

Nutritional Information (per serving): Calories: 250kcal; Fat: 6g; Carbs: 40g; Protein: 12g

Veggie-packed Frittata Feast

Preparation time: 15 minutes

Cooking time: 20 minutes

Servings: 2

Ingredients:

- 4 eggs
- 1/4 cup milk
- 1/2 cup cherry tomatoes, halved
- 1/2 cup spinach, chopped
- 1/4 cup red bell pepper, diced
- 1/4 cup onion, finely chopped
- 1/4 cup feta cheese, crumbled
- Salt and pepper to taste
- Cooking spray

Instructions:

1. Preheat the oven to 350°F (175°C).
2. In a bowl, whisk together the eggs, milk, salt, and pepper.
3. Heat an oven-safe skillet over medium heat, coat with cooking spray.
4. Add onions and bell peppers, sauté until softened.
5. Add cherry tomatoes and spinach, cook until wilted.
6. Pour the egg mixture over the veggies and sprinkle feta cheese on top.
7. Transfer the skillet to the preheated oven and bake for about 15-20 minutes or until the frittata is set.
8. Slice and serve.

Nutritional Information (per serving): Calories: 280kcal; Fat: 20g; Carbs: 8g; Protein: 18g

Quinoa Power Porridge

Preparation time: 5 minutes

Cooking time: 15 minutes

Servings: 2

Ingredients:

- 1/2 cup quinoa, rinsed
- 1 cup almond milk
- 1/2 teaspoon cinnamon
- 1/4 cup sliced almonds
- 1 tablespoon honey
- Fresh berries for topping

Instructions:

1. In a saucepan, combine quinoa and almond milk. Bring to a boil, then reduce heat to low, cover, and simmer for 15 minutes or until quinoa is cooked.
2. Stir in cinnamon and sliced almonds.
3. Divide into bowls and drizzle with honey.
4. Top with fresh berries.

Nutritional Information (per serving): Calories: 300kcal; Fat: 10g; Carbs: 45g; Protein: 8g

High-Protein Blueberry Muffins

Preparation time: 10 minutes

Cooking time: 20 minutes

Servings: 2 (6 muffins each)

Ingredients:

- 1 cup almond flour
- 1/4 cup protein powder
- 1 teaspoon baking powder
- 1/4 teaspoon salt
- 2 eggs
- 1/4 cup almond milk
- 1/4 cup melted coconut oil
- 1/4 cup honey
- 1 cup blueberries

Instructions:

1. Preheat the oven to 350°F (175°C) and line a muffin tin with paper liners.
2. In a bowl, whisk together almond flour, protein powder, baking powder, and salt.
3. In another bowl, beat eggs, then add almond milk, melted coconut oil, and honey.
4. Combine wet and dry ingredients, then fold in blueberries.
5. Spoon the batter into muffin cups and bake for 20 minutes or until a toothpick comes out clean.
6. Allow muffins to cool before serving.

Nutritional Information (per serving - 3 muffins): Calories: 320kcal; Fat: 20g; Carbs: 25g; Protein: 12g

Avocado and Salmon Breakfast Wrap

Preparation time: 10 minutes

Cooking time: 5 minutes

Servings: 2

Ingredients:

- 2 whole wheat tortillas
- 1/2 avocado, sliced
- 4 oz smoked salmon
- 2 eggs, scrambled
- Fresh dill for garnish
- Salt and pepper to taste

Instructions:

1. Warm the tortillas in a dry skillet over medium heat.
2. Spread sliced avocado on each tortilla.
3. Divide scrambled eggs and smoked salmon between the tortillas.
4. Season with salt, pepper, and garnish with fresh dill.
5. Roll up the wraps and serve.

Nutritional Information (per serving): Calories: 350kcal; Fat: 20g; Carbs: 25g; Protein: 18g

Greek Yogurt Parfait with Nutty Granola

Preparation time: 5 minutes

Cooking time: 10 minutes

Servings: 2

Ingredients:

- 2 cups Greek yogurt
- 1 cup mixed berries (strawberries, blueberries, raspberries)
- 1/2 cup nutty granola
- Honey for drizzling

Instructions:

1. In two glasses or bowls, layer Greek yogurt.
2. Add a layer of mixed berries on top of the yogurt.
3. Sprinkle nutty granola over the berries.
4. Repeat the layers.
5. Drizzle honey on the top layer.
6. Serve immediately.

Nutritional Information (per serving): Calories: 300kcal; Fat: 10g; Carbs: 40g; Protein: 15g

Cottage Cheese and Fruit Medley

Preparation time: 5 minutes

Cooking time: 0 minutes

Servings: 2

Ingredients:

- 1 cup cottage cheese
- 1 cup mixed fresh fruit (pineapple, kiwi, mango)
- 1/4 cup sliced almonds
- 1 tablespoon honey

Instructions:

1. In a bowl, spoon cottage cheese.
2. Add mixed fresh fruit on top.
3. Sprinkle sliced almonds over the fruit.
4. Drizzle honey on the mixture.
5. Mix gently and serve.

Nutritional Information (per serving): Calories: 250kcal; Fat: 10g; Carbs: 25g; Protein: 20g

Almond Butter Banana Toast with a Twist

Preparation time: 5 minutes

Cooking time: 5 minutes

Servings: 2

Ingredients:

- 2 slices whole wheat bread
- 2 tablespoons almond butter
- 1 banana, sliced
- 1 tablespoon chia seeds
- Drizzle of honey

Instructions:

1. Toast the whole wheat bread slices.
2. Spread almond butter evenly on each slice.
3. Arrange banana slices on top of the almond butter.
4. Sprinkle chia seeds over the bananas.
5. Drizzle honey over the top.
6. Serve and enjoy.

Nutritional Information (per serving): Calories: 320kcal; Fat: 14g; Carbs: 45g; Protein: 8g

Zesty Breakfast Burrito with Lean Turkey

Preparation time: 15 minutes

Cooking time: 10 minutes

Servings: 2

Ingredients:

- 4 large eggs
- 1/2 cup lean ground turkey
- 1/4 cup diced bell peppers (assorted colors)
- 1/4 cup diced onions
- 1/4 cup shredded cheddar cheese
- 2 whole wheat or spinach tortillas
- Salt and pepper to taste
- Salsa and avocado for topping

Instructions:

1. In a skillet, cook lean ground turkey until fully browned.
2. Add diced bell peppers and onions to the skillet; sauté until vegetables are tender.
3. In a separate bowl, whisk eggs and pour them into the skillet.
4. Scramble eggs with the turkey and veggies until fully cooked.
5. Warm tortillas in the skillet or microwave.
6. Divide the egg and turkey mixture between the tortillas.
7. Top each burrito with shredded cheddar cheese, salsa, and slices of avocado.
8. Fold the tortillas to create burritos.
9. Serve warm.

Nutritional Information (per serving): Calories: 400kcal; Fat: 20g; Carbs: 25g; Protein: 25g

Coconut Flour Waffles with Fresh Berries

Preparation time: 10 minutes

Cooking time: 15 minutes

Servings: 2

Ingredients:

- 1/2 cup coconut flour
- 1 teaspoon baking powder
- 2 large eggs
- 1 cup almond milk
- 1 tablespoon melted coconut oil
- 1 tablespoon honey
- Fresh berries for topping

Instructions:

1. Preheat your waffle iron.
2. In a bowl, whisk together coconut flour and baking powder.
3. In a separate bowl, beat eggs and add almond milk, melted coconut oil, and honey.
4. Combine wet and dry ingredients and mix until smooth.
5. Pour batter onto the preheated waffle iron and cook according to the iron's instructions.
6. Once cooked, transfer waffles to plates.
7. Top with fresh berries and a drizzle of honey.
8. Serve and enjoy.

Nutritional Information (per serving): Calories: 300kcal; Fat: 15g; Carbs: 35g; Protein: 10g

Chapter 4:
Snacks and Drinks

Snacks:

Nutty Trail Mix Crunch

Preparation time: 5 minutes

Cooking time: 10 minutes (toasting nuts, optional)

Servings: 2

Ingredients:

- 1/2 cup almonds
- 1/2 cup walnuts
- 1/4 cup pumpkin seeds
- 1/4 cup dried cranberries
- 1/4 cup dark chocolate chips
- 1/4 teaspoon sea salt (optional)

Instructions:

1. If desired, toast the almonds and walnuts in a dry skillet over medium heat for 5-7 minutes, stirring frequently until fragrant.
2. In a bowl, combine toasted nuts, pumpkin seeds, dried cranberries, and dark chocolate chips.
3. Add sea salt if desired and toss to combine.
4. Let it cool and then store in an airtight container.

Nutritional Information (per serving): Calories: 300kcal; Fat: 24g; Carbs: 18g; Protein: 8g

Crunchy Veggie Sticks with Hummus

Preparation time: 10 minutes

Cooking time: 0 minutes

Servings: 2

Ingredients:

- 2 medium carrots, peeled and cut into sticks
- 2 medium cucumbers, cut into sticks
- 1 bell pepper (any color), sliced
- 1 cup cherry tomatoes, halved
- Hummus for dipping

Instructions:

1. Prepare all vegetables and arrange them on a serving plate.
2. Place hummus in a small bowl at the center of the plate.
3. Serve the crunchy veggie sticks with hummus for dipping.

Nutritional Information (per serving): Calories: 150kcal; Fat: 6g; Carbs: 22g; Protein: 5g

Hard-Boiled Eggs with a Kick

Preparation time: 5 minutes

Cooking time: 10 minutes

Servings: 2

Ingredients:

- 4 large eggs
- 1 teaspoon hot sauce
- Salt and pepper to taste
- Fresh herbs for garnish (optional)

Instructions:

1. Place eggs in a saucepan and cover with water.
2. Bring water to a boil, then reduce heat and simmer for 9-10 minutes.
3. Transfer eggs to an ice bath to cool.
4. Once cooled, peel the eggs and cut them in half.
5. Drizzle hot sauce over each egg half.
6. Season with salt and pepper, and garnish with fresh herbs if desired.

Nutritional Information (per serving): Calories: 140kcal; Fat: 10g; Carbs: 1g; Protein: 12g

Almond and Coconut Energy Bites

Preparation time: 15 minutes

Cooking time: 0 minutes (no baking required)

Servings: 2

Ingredients:

- 1 cup old-fashioned oats
- 1/2 cup almond butter
- 1/3 cup honey
- 1/2 cup shredded coconut
- 1/2 cup chopped almonds
- 1 teaspoon vanilla extract
- Pinch of salt

Instructions:

1. In a large bowl, combine oats, almond butter, honey, shredded coconut, chopped almonds, vanilla extract, and a pinch of salt.
2. Mix until well combined.
3. Take small portions and roll them into bite-sized balls.
4. Place the energy bites on a tray and refrigerate for at least 1 hour before serving.

Nutritional Information (per serving): Calories: 300kcal; Fat: 18g; Carbs: 30g; Protein: 8g

Spicy Roasted Chickpeas Snack

Preparation time: 10 minutes

Cooking time: 30 minutes

Servings: 2

Ingredients:

- 1 can (15 oz) chickpeas, drained and rinsed
- 1 tablespoon olive oil
- 1 teaspoon smoked paprika
- 1/2 teaspoon cayenne pepper
- Salt to taste

Instructions:

1. Preheat the oven to 400°F (200°C).
2. Pat dry the chickpeas with a paper towel.
3. In a bowl, toss chickpeas with olive oil, smoked paprika, cayenne pepper, and salt.
4. Spread the chickpeas on a baking sheet in a single layer.
5. Roast in the oven for 30 minutes or until crispy, shaking the pan occasionally.
6. Let them cool before serving.

Nutritional Information (per serving): Calories: 220kcal; Fat: 7g; Carbs: 33g; Protein: 8g

Avocado Salsa with Whole Grain Crackers

Preparation time: 10 minutes

Cooking time: 0 minutes

Servings: 2

Ingredients:

- 1 ripe avocado, diced
- 1/2 cup cherry tomatoes, halved
- 1/4 cup red onion, finely chopped
- 1/4 cup fresh cilantro, chopped
- 1 jalapeño, seeds removed and finely chopped
- Juice of 1 lime
- Salt and pepper to taste
- Whole grain crackers for serving

Instructions:

1. In a bowl, combine diced avocado, cherry tomatoes, red onion, cilantro, jalapeño, lime juice, salt, and pepper.
2. Mix gently until well combined.
3. Serve the avocado salsa with whole grain crackers.

Nutritional Information (per serving): Calories: 250kcal; Fat: 18g; Carbs: 20g; Protein: 4g

Cucumber Slices with Tzatziki Dip

Preparation time: 15 minutes

Cooking time: 0 minutes

Servings: 2

Ingredients:

- 1 cucumber, thinly sliced
- 1 cup Greek yogurt
- 1/2 cup cucumber, finely diced
- 1 tablespoon fresh dill, chopped
- 1 clove garlic, minced
- 1 tablespoon lemon juice
- Salt and pepper to taste

Instructions:

1. In a bowl, combine Greek yogurt, diced cucumber, fresh dill, minced garlic, lemon juice, salt, and pepper.
2. Mix until well combined.
3. Arrange the cucumber slices on a plate and serve with the tzatziki dip.

Nutritional Information (per serving): Calories: 90kcal; Fat: 3g; Carbs: 10g; Protein: 6g

Guacamole-Stuffed Cherry Tomatoes

Preparation time: 20 minutes

Cooking time: 0 minutes

Servings: 2

Ingredients:

- 1 cup cherry tomatoes
- 2 ripe avocados
- 1/4 cup red onion, finely chopped
- 1/4 cup cilantro, chopped
- 1 lime, juiced
- Salt and pepper to taste

Instructions:

1. Cut the tops off the cherry tomatoes and scoop out the seeds to create small cups.
2. In a bowl, mash the ripe avocados.
3. Add chopped red onion, cilantro, lime juice, salt, and pepper to the mashed avocados. Mix well.
4. Spoon the guacamole mixture into the hollowed cherry tomatoes.
5. Arrange on a serving platter and garnish with additional cilantro if desired.

Nutritional Information (per serving): Calories: 180kcal; Fat: 14g; Carbs: 12g; Protein: 3g

Drinks:

Greek Yogurt and Berry Smoothie

Preparation time: 5 minutes

Cooking time: 0 minutes

Servings: 2

Ingredients:

- 1 cup Greek yogurt
- 1 cup mixed berries (strawberries, blueberries, raspberries)
- 1 banana
- 1 tablespoon honey
- 1/2 cup almond milk
- Ice cubes (optional)

Instructions:

1. In a blender, combine Greek yogurt, mixed berries, banana, honey, and almond milk.
2. Blend until smooth.
3. Add ice cubes if desired and blend again.
4. Pour into glasses and serve.

Nutritional Information (per serving): Calories: 220kcal; Fat: 3g; Carbs: 40g; Protein: 12g

Green Tea Infusion for Antioxidant Boost

Preparation time: 5 minutes

Cooking time: 5 minutes

Servings: 2

Ingredients:
- 2 green tea bags
- 2 cups hot water
- 1 tablespoon honey
- Lemon slices (optional)
- Fresh mint leaves (optional)

Instructions:
1. Steep the green tea bags in hot water for 3-5 minutes.
2. Remove the tea bags and stir in honey until dissolved.
3. Allow the tea to cool.
4. Refrigerate until chilled.
5. Serve over ice with lemon slices and fresh mint if desired.

Nutritional Information (per serving): Calories: 10kcal; Carbs: 3g; Sugar: 2g

Fresh Fruit Kabobs with Mint Yogurt Dip

Preparation time: 15 minutes

Cooking time: 0 minutes

Servings: 2

Ingredients:
- Assorted fresh fruits (strawberries, pineapple, grapes, melon)
- 1 cup Greek yogurt
- 1 tablespoon honey
- Fresh mint leaves for garnish

Instructions:
1. Cut the fresh fruits into bite-sized pieces.
2. Thread the fruit pieces onto skewers.
3. In a bowl, mix Greek yogurt and honey.
4. Serve the fruit kabobs with the mint yogurt dip.
5. Garnish with fresh mint leaves.

Nutritional Information (per serving): Calories: 180kcal; Fat: 1g; Carbs: 35g; Protein: 10g

Iced Herbal Infusion with Citrus Twist

Preparation time: 10 minutes

Cooking time: 0 minutes

Servings: 2

Ingredients:

- 2 herbal tea bags (e.g., chamomile, peppermint)
- 2 cups hot water
- 1 orange, sliced
- 1 lemon, sliced
- Fresh mint leaves
- Ice cubes

Instructions:

1. Steep the herbal tea bags in hot water for 5-7 minutes.
2. Allow the tea to cool and then refrigerate until chilled.
3. Fill glasses with ice cubes and pour the herbal tea over the ice.
4. Add slices of orange and lemon.
5. Garnish with fresh mint leaves.

Nutritional Information (per serving): Calories: 5kcal; Carbs: 1g; Sugar: 0g

Berry Blast Protein Shake

Preparation time: 5 minutes

Cooking time: 0 minutes

Servings: 2

Ingredients:

- 1 cup mixed berries (strawberries, blueberries, raspberries)
- 1 scoop vanilla protein powder
- 1 cup almond milk
- 1 tablespoon almond butter
- Ice cubes

Instructions:

1. In a blender, combine mixed berries, protein powder, almond milk, and almond butter.
2. Blend until smooth.
3. Add ice cubes and blend again until desired consistency.
4. Pour into glasses and serve.

Nutritional Information (per serving): Calories: 220kcal; Fat: 8g; Carbs: 15g; Protein: 20g

Minty Matcha Latte

Preparation time: 5 minutes

Cooking time: 5 minutes

Servings: 2

Ingredients:

- 2 teaspoons matcha powder
- 2 cups almond milk
- 1 tablespoon honey
- Fresh mint leaves for garnish

Instructions:

1. In a saucepan, heat almond milk until warm but not boiling.
2. Whisk in matcha powder until well combined.
3. Stir in honey until dissolved.
4. Pour into mugs and garnish with fresh mint leaves.

Nutritional Information (per serving): Calories: 80kcal; Carbs: 15g; Sugar: 10g

Tropical Pineapple Coconut Smoothie

Preparation time: 8 minutes

Cooking time: 0 minutes

Servings: 2

Ingredients:

- 1 cup pineapple chunks
- 1/2 cup coconut milk
- 1/2 cup Greek yogurt
- 1 tablespoon chia seeds
- Ice cubes

Instructions:

1. In a blender, combine pineapple chunks, coconut milk, Greek yogurt, and chia seeds.
2. Blend until smooth.
3. Add ice cubes and blend again.
4. Pour into glasses and serve.

Nutritional Information (per serving): Calories: 180kcal; Fat: 8g; Carbs: 20g; Protein: 8g

Refreshing Cucumber Mint Cooler

Preparation time: 10 minutes

Cooking time: 0 minutes

Servings: 2

Ingredients:

- 1 cucumber, sliced
- 1/4 cup fresh mint leaves
- 1 tablespoon honey
- 1 tablespoon lime juice
- Sparkling water
- Ice cubes

Instructions:

1. In a pitcher, muddle cucumber slices, mint leaves, honey, and lime juice.
2. Fill the pitcher with ice cubes and top with sparkling water.
3. Stir gently and serve.

Nutritional Information (per serving): Calories: 20kcal; Carbs: 5g; Sugar: 3g

Chapter 5: Beef, Pork, and Poultry Recipes

Grilled Lemon-Herb Chicken Breast

Preparation time: 10 minutes

Cooking time: 15 minutes

Servings: 2

Ingredients:

- 2 boneless, skinless chicken breasts
- 2 tablespoons olive oil
- 1 tablespoon lemon juice
- 1 teaspoon dried thyme
- 1 teaspoon dried rosemary
- Salt and pepper to taste

Instructions:

1. In a bowl, mix olive oil, lemon juice, thyme, rosemary, salt, and pepper.
2. Coat chicken breasts with the marinade and let them marinate for at least 30 minutes.
3. Preheat the grill and cook the chicken for about 7-8 minutes per side or until fully cooked.
4. Serve hot.

Nutritional Information (per serving): Calories: 250kcal; Fat: 14g; Carbs: 1g; Protein: 30g

Savory Garlic and Rosemary Beef Skewers

Preparation time: 15 minutes

Cooking time: 10 minutes

Servings: 2

Ingredients:

- 1 pound beef sirloin, cut into cubes
- 2 tablespoons olive oil
- 3 cloves garlic, minced
- 1 tablespoon fresh rosemary, chopped
- Salt and pepper to taste

Instructions:

1. In a bowl, mix olive oil, minced garlic, chopped rosemary, salt, and pepper.
2. Thread beef cubes onto skewers and brush with the garlic-rosemary mixture.
3. Grill for about 4-5 minutes per side or until desired doneness.
4. Serve immediately.

Nutritional Information (per serving): Calories: 400kcal; Fat: 28g; Carbs: 1g; Protein: 35g

Mediterranean Turkey Meatballs

Preparation time: 20 minutes

Cooking time: 20 minutes

Servings: 2

Ingredients:

- 1/2 pound ground turkey
- 1/4 cup breadcrumbs
- 1/4 cup feta cheese, crumbled
- 1/4 cup black olives, chopped
- 1 teaspoon dried oregano
- Salt and pepper to taste

Instructions:

1. Preheat the oven to 375°F (190°C).
2. In a bowl, combine ground turkey, breadcrumbs, feta cheese, black olives, oregano, salt, and pepper.
3. Form the mixture into meatballs and place them on a baking sheet.
4. Bake for about 18-20 minutes or until cooked through.
5. Serve with your favorite sauce.

Nutritional Information (per serving): Calories: 320kcal; Fat: 20g; Carbs: 10g; Protein: 25g

Citrus-Marinated Grilled Pork Chops

Preparation time: 15 minutes

Cooking time: 12 minutes

Servings: 2

Ingredients:

- 2 pork chops
- 1/4 cup orange juice
- 2 tablespoons lime juice
- 1 tablespoon honey
- 1 teaspoon cumin
- Salt and pepper to taste

Instructions:

1. In a bowl, whisk together orange juice, lime juice, honey, cumin, salt, and pepper.
2. Marinate pork chops in the citrus mixture for at least 30 minutes.
3. Preheat the grill and cook pork chops for about 6 minutes per side or until fully cooked.
4. Let them rest for a few minutes before serving.

Nutritional Information (per serving): Calories: 300kcal; Fat: 15g; Carbs: 10g; Protein: 25g

Spicy Sriracha Chicken Stir-Fry

Preparation time: 15 minutes

Cooking time: 10 minutes

Servings: 2

Ingredients:

- 1 pound chicken breast, thinly sliced
- 2 tablespoons soy sauce
- 1 tablespoon Sriracha sauce
- 1 tablespoon honey
- 1 tablespoon vegetable oil
- 2 cloves garlic, minced
- 1 bell pepper, sliced
- 1 cup broccoli florets
- Cooked brown rice for serving

Instructions:

1. In a bowl, mix soy sauce, Sriracha sauce, and honey.
2. Heat vegetable oil in a wok or skillet and sauté minced garlic until fragrant.
3. Add sliced chicken and stir-fry until browned.
4. Add bell pepper and broccoli, continuing to stir-fry until vegetables are tender.
5. Pour the sauce over the stir-fry and toss until well-coated.
6. Serve over cooked brown rice.

Nutritional Information (per serving): Calories: 400kcal; Fat: 15g; Carbs: 30g; Protein: 35g

Lean Beef and Vegetable Stuffed Peppers

Preparation time: 20 minutes

Cooking time: 25 minutes

Servings: 2

Ingredients:

- 2 large bell peppers, halved and seeds removed
- 1/2 pound lean ground beef
- 1 cup cauliflower rice
- 1/2 cup black beans, drained and rinsed
- 1/2 cup corn kernels
- 1/2 cup salsa
- 1 teaspoon cumin
- Salt and pepper to taste
- Shredded cheese for topping (optional)

Instructions:

1. Preheat the oven to 375°F (190°C).
2. In a skillet, brown the ground beef. Drain excess fat.
3. Stir in cauliflower rice, black beans, corn, salsa, cumin, salt, and pepper.
4. Spoon the mixture into halved bell peppers.
5. Bake for about 20-25 minutes or until peppers are tender.
6. Top with shredded cheese if desired and bake for an additional 5 minutes.

Nutritional Information (per serving): Calories: 250kcal; Fat: 15g; Carbs: 30g; Protein: 25g

Tangy Teriyaki Chicken Thighs

Preparation time: 15 minutes

Cooking time: 20 minutes

Servings: 2

Ingredients:

- 4 bone-in, skinless chicken thighs
- 1/4 cup soy sauce
- 2 tablespoons honey
- 1 tablespoon rice vinegar
- 1 tablespoon minced ginger
- 2 cloves garlic, minced
- Sesame seeds and green onions for garnish

Instructions:

1. Preheat the oven to 400°F (200°C).
2. In a bowl, whisk together soy sauce, honey, rice vinegar, minced ginger, and minced garlic.
3. Place chicken thighs in a baking dish and pour the teriyaki sauce over them.
4. Bake for about 20 minutes or until chicken is fully cooked.
5. Garnish with sesame seeds and chopped green onions before serving.

Nutritional Information (per serving): Calories: 400kcal; Fat: 20g; Carbs: 20g; Protein: 30g

Zesty Lime and Cilantro Turkey Burgers

Preparation time: 15 minutes

Cooking time: 15 minutes

Servings: 2

Ingredients:

- 1/2 pound ground turkey
- 1/4 cup breadcrumbs
- 1/4 cup fresh cilantro, chopped
- 1 tablespoon lime juice
- 1 teaspoon ground cumin
- Salt and pepper to taste
- Whole wheat burger buns and toppings of choice

Instructions:

1. In a bowl, combine ground turkey, breadcrumbs, chopped cilantro, lime juice, cumin, salt, and pepper.
2. Form the mixture into burger patties.
3. Grill or pan-sear the turkey burgers for about 6-8 minutes per side or until fully cooked.
4. Serve on whole wheat buns with your favorite toppings.

Nutritional Information (per serving): Calories: 300kcal; Fat: 10g; Carbs: 25g; Protein: 25g

Slow-Cooked Italian Herb Pulled Pork

Preparation time: 15 minutes

Cooking time: 6-8 hours (slow cooker)

Servings: 2

Ingredients:

- 1 pound pork shoulder, trimmed of excess fat
- 1 cup tomato sauce
- 1/4 cup balsamic vinegar
- 1 tablespoon Italian seasoning
- 1 teaspoon garlic powder
- Salt and pepper to taste
- Whole wheat buns for serving

Instructions:

1. Season the pork shoulder with salt, pepper, and garlic powder.
2. In a slow cooker, combine pork shoulder, tomato sauce, balsamic vinegar, and Italian seasoning.
3. Cook on low for 6-8 hours until the pork is tender and easily shredded.
4. Shred the pork using two forks and mix with the cooking juices.
5. Serve on whole wheat buns.

Nutritional Information (per serving): Calories: 350kcal; Fat: 15g; Carbs: 20g; Protein: 30g

Sesame-Ginger Glazed Chicken Drumsticks

Preparation time: 15 minutes

Cooking time: 35 minutes

Servings: 2

Ingredients:

- 8 chicken drumsticks
- 1/4 cup soy sauce
- 2 tablespoons honey
- 1 tablespoon sesame oil
- 1 tablespoon rice vinegar
- 1 teaspoon minced ginger
- 2 cloves garlic, minced
- Sesame seeds and chopped green onions for garnish

Instructions:

1. Preheat the oven to 425°F (220°C).
2. In a bowl, whisk together soy sauce, honey, sesame oil, rice vinegar, minced ginger, and minced garlic.
3. Place chicken drumsticks in a baking dish and pour the glaze over them.
4. Bake for about 30-35 minutes or until chicken is fully cooked.
5. Garnish with sesame seeds and chopped green onions before serving.

Nutritional Information (per serving): Calories: 400kcal; Fat: 20g; Carbs: 15g; Protein: 30g

Chipotle Lime Grilled Steak Strips

Preparation time: 10 minutes (plus marinating time)

Cooking time: 10 minutes

Servings: 2

Ingredients:

- 1/2 pound flank steak, thinly sliced
- 2 tablespoons olive oil
- 1 tablespoon lime juice
- 1 teaspoon chipotle powder
- 1 teaspoon garlic powder
- Salt and pepper to taste
- Fresh cilantro for garnish

Instructions:

1. In a bowl, whisk together olive oil, lime juice, chipotle powder, garlic powder, salt, and pepper.
2. Marinate the sliced flank steak in the mixture for at least 30 minutes.
3. Preheat the grill or grill pan over medium-high heat.
4. Grill the steak strips for about 3-4 minutes per side or to your desired doneness.
5. Garnish with fresh cilantro before serving.

Nutritional Information (per serving): Calories: 300kcal; Fat: 20g; Carbs: 2g; Protein: 25g

Chapter 6:
Fish and Seafood Recipes

Lemon-Garlic Grilled Salmon

Preparation time: 10 minutes (plus marinating time)

Cooking time: 10 minutes

Servings: 2

Ingredients:

- 2 salmon fillets
- 2 tablespoons olive oil
- 2 tablespoons fresh lemon juice
- 2 cloves garlic, minced
- 1 teaspoon dried oregano
- Salt and black pepper to taste
- Lemon wedges for garnish

Instructions:

1. In a bowl, mix olive oil, lemon juice, minced garlic, dried oregano, salt, and black pepper.
2. Marinate the salmon fillets in the mixture for at least 30 minutes.
3. Preheat the grill to medium-high heat.
4. Grill the salmon for about 4-5 minutes per side or until cooked through.
5. Garnish with lemon wedges before serving.

Nutritional Information (per serving): Calories: 350kcal; Fat: 24g; Carbs: 1g; Protein: 30g

Spicy Shrimp and Zucchini Noodles

Preparation time: 15 minutes

Cooking time: 10 minutes

Servings: 2

Ingredients:

- 1 pound large shrimp, peeled and deveined
- 2 medium zucchinis, spiralized into noodles
- 2 tablespoons olive oil
- 2 cloves garlic, minced
- 1 teaspoon red pepper flakes
- Salt and black pepper to taste
- Fresh parsley for garnish

Instructions:

1. In a skillet, heat olive oil over medium heat and sauté minced garlic until fragrant.
2. Add shrimp to the skillet and cook for 2-3 minutes per side or until opaque.
3. Add zucchini noodles, red pepper flakes, salt, and black pepper. Cook for an additional 3-4 minutes.
4. Garnish with fresh parsley before serving.

Nutritional Information (per serving): Calories: 280kcal; Fat: 16g; Carbs: 8g; Protein: 25g

Baked Cod with Herbed Quinoa

Preparation time: 15 minutes

Cooking time: 20 minutes

Servings: 2

Ingredients:

- 2 cod fillets
- 1 cup quinoa, cooked
- 2 tablespoons olive oil
- 1 tablespoon fresh lemon juice
- 1 teaspoon dried thyme
- 1 teaspoon dried rosemary
- Salt and black pepper to taste
- Fresh dill for garnish

Instructions:

1. Preheat the oven to 400°F (200°C).
2. Place cod fillets on a baking sheet and drizzle with olive oil and lemon juice.
3. Sprinkle dried thyme, dried rosemary, salt, and black pepper over the cod.
4. Bake for 15-20 minutes or until the cod is flaky.
5. Serve over herbed quinoa and garnish with fresh dill.

Nutritional Information (per serving): Calories: 380kcal; Fat: 16g; Carbs: 28g; Protein: 30g

Teriyaki Glazed Tuna Steaks

Preparation time: 15 minutes (plus marinating time)

Cooking time: 8 minutes

Servings: 2

Ingredients:

- 2 tuna steaks
- 1/4 cup soy sauce
- 2 tablespoons honey
- 1 tablespoon rice vinegar
- 1 teaspoon sesame oil
- 2 cloves garlic, minced
- 1 teaspoon grated ginger
- Sesame seeds and green onions for garnish

Instructions:

1. In a bowl, whisk together soy sauce, honey, rice vinegar, sesame oil, minced garlic, and grated ginger.
2. Marinate the tuna steaks in the mixture for at least 30 minutes.
3. Preheat the grill to medium-high heat.
4. Grill the tuna steaks for about 4 minutes per side or until desired doneness.
5. Garnish with sesame seeds and chopped green onions before serving.

Nutritional Information (per serving): Calories: 280kcal; Fat: 12g; Carbs: 15g; Protein: 30g

Citrus Herb Grilled Sea Bass

Preparation time: 10 minutes (plus marinating time)

Cooking time: 10 minutes

Servings: 2

Ingredients:

- 2 sea bass fillets
- 1/4 cup olive oil
- Zest and juice of 1 lemon
- 2 tablespoons chopped fresh herbs (such as parsley, thyme, or rosemary)
- Salt and black pepper to taste
- Lemon wedges for serving

Instructions:

1. In a bowl, combine olive oil, lemon zest, lemon juice, chopped herbs, salt, and black pepper.
2. Marinate the sea bass fillets in the mixture for at least 15 minutes.
3. Preheat the grill to medium heat.
4. Grill the sea bass for about 4-5 minutes per side or until the fish flakes easily.
5. Serve with lemon wedges.

Nutritional Information (per serving): Calories: 320kcal; Fat: 22g; Carbs: 1g; Protein: 28g

Garlic Butter Shrimp Skewers

Preparation time: 10 minutes (plus marinating time)

Cooking time: 6 minutes

Servings: 2

Ingredients:

- 1/2 pound large shrimp, peeled and deveined
- 2 tablespoons melted butter
- 3 cloves garlic, minced
- 1 tablespoon chopped fresh parsley
- 1 teaspoon paprika
- Salt and black pepper to taste
- Lemon wedges for serving

Instructions:

1. In a bowl, mix melted butter, minced garlic, chopped parsley, paprika, salt, and black pepper.
2. Marinate the shrimp in the mixture for at least 15 minutes.
3. Thread the shrimp onto skewers.
4. Preheat the grill to medium-high heat.
5. Grill the shrimp skewers for about 3 minutes per side or until they turn pink.
6. Serve with lemon wedges.

Nutritional Information (per serving): Calories: 220kcal; Fat: 15g; Carbs: 2g; Protein: 20g

Coconut-Crusted Tilapia Bites

Preparation time: 15 minutes

Cooking time: 8 minutes

Servings: 2

Ingredients:

- 1/2 pound tilapia fillets, cut into bite-sized pieces
- 1/2 cup shredded coconut
- 1/4 cup almond flour
- 1 teaspoon paprika
- 1/2 teaspoon garlic powder
- 1/4 cup coconut milk
- 1 egg, beaten
- Coconut oil for frying

Instructions:

1. In a bowl, combine shredded coconut, almond flour, paprika, and garlic powder.
2. Dip each tilapia bite into coconut milk, then coat with the coconut mixture.
3. Heat coconut oil in a skillet over medium heat.
4. Fry the coated tilapia bites for about 3-4 minutes per side or until golden brown.
5. Drain on paper towels before serving.

Nutritional Information (per serving): Calories: 280kcal; Fat: 20g; Carbs: 8g; Protein: 20g

Cajun-Style Blackened Catfish

Preparation time: 10 minutes (plus marinating time)

Cooking time: 8 minutes

Servings: 2

Ingredients:

- 2 catfish fillets
- 2 teaspoons Cajun seasoning
- 1 teaspoon paprika
- 1/2 teaspoon garlic powder
- 1/2 teaspoon onion powder
- 1/2 teaspoon thyme
- 1/4 teaspoon cayenne pepper
- 2 tablespoons olive oil
- Lemon wedges for serving

Instructions:

1. In a bowl, mix Cajun seasoning, paprika, garlic powder, onion powder, thyme, and cayenne pepper.
2. Rub the catfish fillets with the spice mixture, ensuring an even coating.
3. Heat olive oil in a skillet over medium-high heat.
4. Cook the catfish for about 4 minutes per side or until the edges are crispy.
5. Serve with lemon wedges.

Nutritional Information (per serving): 240kcal; Fat: 16g; Carbs: 2g; Protein: 22g

Sesame Ginger Marinated Scallops

Preparation time: 15 minutes (plus marinating time)

Cooking time: 5 minutes

Servings: 2

Ingredients:

- 1/2 pound scallops
- 2 tablespoons soy sauce
- 1 tablespoon sesame oil
- 1 tablespoon rice vinegar
- 1 tablespoon grated ginger
- 2 cloves garlic, minced
- 1 tablespoon chopped green onions
- Sesame seeds for garnish

Instructions:

1. In a bowl, whisk together soy sauce, sesame oil, rice vinegar, grated ginger, minced garlic, and green onions.
2. Marinate the scallops in the mixture for at least 30 minutes.
3. Heat a skillet over medium-high heat.
4. Cook the scallops for about 2 minutes per side or until they are opaque.
5. Garnish with sesame seeds before serving.

Nutritional Information (per serving): 180kcal; Fat: 9g; Carbs: 4g; Protein: 20g

Mediterranean Herb Baked Trout

Preparation time: 10 minutes (plus marinating time)

Cooking time: 15 minutes

Servings: 2

Ingredients:

- 2 trout fillets
- 2 tablespoons olive oil
- 1 teaspoon dried oregano
- 1 teaspoon dried thyme
- 1 teaspoon dried rosemary
- 2 cloves garlic, minced
- Lemon wedges for serving

Instructions:

1. Preheat the oven to 375°F (190°C).
2. In a bowl, mix olive oil, dried oregano, dried thyme, dried rosemary, and minced garlic.
3. Rub the trout fillets with the herb mixture, ensuring an even coating.
4. Marinate the trout for at least 15 minutes.
5. Place the fillets on a baking sheet and bake for about 15 minutes or until the fish flakes easily.
6. Serve with lemon wedges.

Nutritional Information (per serving): 280kcal; Fat: 20g; Carbs: 0g; Protein: 24g

Lime Cilantro Grilled Swordfish

Preparation time: 15 minutes (plus marinating time)

Cooking time: 8 minutes

Servings: 2

Ingredients:

- 2 swordfish steaks
- Juice of 2 limes
- 2 tablespoons chopped cilantro
- 1 tablespoon olive oil
- 1 teaspoon cumin
- 1/2 teaspoon chili powder
- Salt and black pepper to taste

Instructions:

1. In a bowl, combine lime juice, chopped cilantro, olive oil, cumin, chili powder, salt, and black pepper.
2. Marinate the swordfish steaks in the mixture for at least 30 minutes.
3. Preheat the grill to medium-high heat.
4. Grill the swordfish for about 4 minutes per side or until the fish is opaque.
5. Serve immediately.

Nutritional Information (per serving): 320kcal; Fat: 20g; Carbs: 2g; Protein: 30g

Chapter 7:
Pasta and Soups

Whole Wheat Penne with Roasted Vegetables

Preparation time: 15 minutes

Cooking time: 25 minutes

Servings: 2

Ingredients:

- 2 cups whole wheat penne pasta
- 1 zucchini, diced
- 1 red bell pepper, sliced
- 1 yellow bell pepper, sliced
- 1 red onion, sliced
- 2 tablespoons olive oil
- 1 teaspoon dried oregano
- 1 teaspoon dried basil
- Salt and black pepper to taste
- Grated Parmesan cheese for garnish

Instructions:

1. Preheat the oven to 425°F (220°C).
2. Toss zucchini, red bell pepper, yellow bell pepper, and red onion with olive oil, dried oregano, dried basil, salt, and black pepper.
3. Spread the vegetables on a baking sheet and roast for about 20 minutes, stirring occasionally.
4. Cook whole wheat penne according to package instructions.
5. Combine roasted vegetables with cooked penne.
6. Garnish with grated Parmesan cheese before serving.

Nutritional Information (per serving): 450kcal; Fat: 10g; Carbs: 80g; Protein: 12

Turmeric Infused Lentil Soup

Preparation time: 15 minutes

Cooking time: 30 minutes

Servings: 2

Ingredients:

- 1 cup dried lentils, rinsed
- 1 carrot, diced
- 1 celery stalk, diced
- 1 onion, chopped
- 2 cloves garlic, minced
- 1 teaspoon turmeric
- 1 teaspoon cumin
- 4 cups vegetable broth
- Salt and black pepper to taste
- Fresh cilantro for garnish

Instructions:

1. In a pot, combine lentils, carrot, celery, onion, garlic, turmeric, cumin, and vegetable broth.
2. Bring to a boil, then reduce heat and simmer for about 25-30 minutes or until lentils are tender.
3. Season with salt and black pepper.
4. Garnish with fresh cilantro before serving.

Nutritional Information (per serving): 350kcal; Fat: 2g; Carbs: 60g; Protein: 20g

Zucchini Noodles with Turkey Bolognese

Preparation time: 15 minutes

Cooking time: 25 minutes

Servings: 2

Ingredients:

- 2 medium zucchinis, spiralized
- 1 pound ground turkey
- 1 onion, chopped
- 2 cloves garlic, minced
- 1 can (14 oz) crushed tomatoes
- 1 teaspoon dried oregano
- 1 teaspoon dried basil
- Salt and black pepper to taste
- Fresh parsley for garnish

Instructions:

1. In a skillet, cook ground turkey until browned.
2. Add chopped onion and minced garlic, cooking until onion is soft.
3. Stir in crushed tomatoes, dried oregano, dried basil, salt, and black pepper. Simmer for 15 minutes.
4. Spiralize zucchinis into noodles.
5. Serve turkey bolognese over zucchini noodles.
6. Garnish with fresh parsley.

Nutritional Information (per serving): 400kcal; Fat: 20g; Carbs: 20g; Protein: 30g

Roasted Red Pepper and Tomato Soup

Preparation time: 15 minutes

Cooking time: 35 minutes

Servings: 2

Ingredients:

- 2 red bell peppers, roasted and peeled
- 1 can (14 oz) diced tomatoes
- 1 onion, chopped
- 2 cloves garlic, minced
- 2 cups vegetable broth
- 1 teaspoon paprika
- 1/2 teaspoon cayenne pepper (optional)
- Salt and black pepper to taste
- Greek yogurt for garnish

Instructions:

1. Roast red bell peppers until the skin is charred, then peel and chop.
2. In a pot, combine roasted red peppers, diced tomatoes, chopped onion, minced garlic, vegetable broth, paprika, and cayenne pepper.
3. Bring to a simmer and cook for about 30 minutes.
4. Blend the soup until smooth.
5. Season with salt and black pepper.
6. Serve with a dollop of Greek yogurt.

Nutritional Information (per serving): 250kcal; Fat: 3g; Carbs: 50g; Protein: 5g

Spinach and Mushroom Quinoa Risotto

Preparation time: 15 minutes

Cooking time: 25 minutes

Servings: 2

Ingredients:

- 1 cup quinoa
- 2 cups vegetable broth
- 1 tablespoon olive oil
- 1 onion, chopped
- 2 cloves garlic, minced
- 1 cup sliced mushrooms
- 2 cups baby spinach
- 1/4 cup grated Parmesan cheese
- Salt and black pepper to taste

Instructions:

1. Rinse quinoa under cold water.
2. In a pot, bring vegetable broth to a simmer.
3. In a skillet, heat olive oil and sauté chopped onion until soft.
4. Add minced garlic and sliced mushrooms, cooking until mushrooms are tender.
5. Stir in quinoa and cook for 1-2 minutes.
6. Begin adding simmering vegetable broth, one ladle at a time, stirring frequently until absorbed.
7. Continue until quinoa is cooked and creamy.
8. Fold in baby spinach until wilted.
9. Stir in grated Parmesan cheese.
10. Season with salt and black pepper before serving.

Nutritional Information (per serving): 400kcal; Fat: 12g; Carbs: 60g; Protein: 15g

Thai Coconut Curry Shrimp Soup

Preparation time: 20 minutes

Cooking time: 25 minutes

Servings: 2

Ingredients:

- 8 oz shrimp, peeled and deveined
- 1 tablespoon coconut oil
- 1 onion, chopped
- 2 cloves garlic, minced
- 1 tablespoon red curry paste
- 1 can (14 oz) coconut milk
- 2 cups chicken broth
- 1 carrot, sliced
- 1 bell pepper, sliced
- 1 tablespoon fish sauce
- 1 tablespoon lime juice
- Fresh cilantro for garnish

Instructions:

1. In a pot, heat coconut oil and sauté chopped onion until translucent.
2. Add minced garlic and red curry paste, cooking for 1-2 minutes.
3. Pour in coconut milk and chicken broth.
4. Add sliced carrot and bell pepper, simmering until vegetables are tender.
5. Stir in shrimp, fish sauce, and lime juice, cooking until shrimp are opaque.
6. Garnish with fresh cilantro before serving.

Nutritional Information (per serving): 450kcal; Fat: 35g; Carbs: 15g; Protein: 25g

Spaghetti Squash Carbonara

Preparation time: 10 minutes

Cooking time: 40 minutes

Servings: 2

Ingredients:

- 1 medium spaghetti squash, halved and seeds removed
- 4 slices turkey bacon, chopped
- 2 cloves garlic, minced
- 2 large eggs
- 1/2 cup grated Parmesan cheese
- Salt and black pepper to taste
- Fresh parsley for garnish

Instructions:

1. Preheat the oven to 400°F (200°C).
2. Place spaghetti squash halves on a baking sheet, cut side down. Roast for about 30-40 minutes or until tender.
3. In a skillet, cook chopped turkey bacon until crispy.
4. Add minced garlic to the skillet, cooking for 1-2 minutes.
5. In a bowl, whisk together eggs and grated Parmesan cheese.
6. Scrape the spaghetti squash into the skillet, mixing with bacon and garlic.
7. Pour the egg and cheese mixture over the squash, tossing quickly to combine.
8. Season with salt and black pepper.
9. Garnish with fresh parsley before serving.

Nutritional Information (per serving): 350kcal; Fat: 22g; Carbs: 20g; Protein: 18g

Spicy Cauliflower and Chickpea Soup

Preparation time: 15 minutes

Cooking time: 30 minutes

Servings: 2

Ingredients:

- 1/2 head cauliflower, chopped
- 1 can (14 oz) chickpeas, drained and rinsed
- 1 onion, chopped
- 2 cloves garlic, minced
- 4 cups vegetable broth
- 1 teaspoon cumin
- 1/2 teaspoon smoked paprika
- 1/4 teaspoon cayenne pepper
- Salt and black pepper to taste
- Greek yogurt for garnish

Instructions:

1. In a pot, combine chopped cauliflower, chickpeas, chopped onion, minced garlic, vegetable broth, cumin, smoked paprika, and cayenne pepper.
2. Bring to a boil, then reduce heat and simmer for about 25-30 minutes.
3. Blend the soup until smooth.
4. Season with salt and black pepper.
5. Serve with a dollop of Greek yogurt.

Nutritional Information (per serving): 300kcal; Fat: 8g; Carbs: 45g; Protein: 12g

Eggplant and Tomato Linguine

Preparation time: 15 minutes

Cooking time: 20 minutes

Servings: 2

Ingredients:

- 4 oz linguine pasta
- 1 medium eggplant, diced
- 2 cups cherry tomatoes, halved
- 2 cloves garlic, minced
- 2 tablespoons olive oil
- 1/4 cup fresh basil, chopped
- Salt and black pepper to taste
- Grated Parmesan cheese for garnish

Instructions:

1. Cook linguine according to package instructions.
2. In a skillet, sauté diced eggplant in olive oil until golden brown.
3. Add halved cherry tomatoes and minced garlic, cooking for an additional 2-3 minutes.
4. Toss the cooked linguine into the skillet, mixing well.
5. Season with salt and black pepper.
6. Garnish with fresh basil and grated Parmesan cheese before serving.

Nutritional Information (per serving): 400kcal; Fat: 12g; Carbs: 65g; Protein: 10g

Lemon Dill Chicken and Orzo Soup

Preparation time: 15 minutes

Cooking time: 25 minutes

Servings: 2

Ingredients:

- 8 oz chicken breast, cooked and shredded
- 1/2 cup orzo pasta
- 1 carrot, sliced
- 1 celery stalk, sliced
- 1 onion, chopped
- 2 cloves garlic, minced
- 4 cups chicken broth
- Zest and juice of 1 lemon
- 1 teaspoon dried dill
- Salt and black pepper to taste
- Fresh dill for garnish

Instructions:

1. In a pot, combine shredded chicken, orzo pasta, sliced carrot, sliced celery, chopped onion, minced garlic, chicken broth, lemon zest, lemon juice, and dried dill.
2. Bring to a simmer and cook for about 20-25 minutes.
3. Season with salt and black pepper.
4. Garnish with fresh dill before serving.

Nutritional Information (per serving): 350kcal; Fat: 10g; Carbs: 30g; Protein: 30g

Chapter 8:
Vegan and Vegetarian

Quinoa and Black Bean Stuffed Bell Peppers

Preparation time: 15 minutes

Cooking time: 30 minutes

Servings: 2

Ingredients

- 1/2 cup quinoa, cooked
- 1 can (14 oz) black beans, drained and rinsed
- 2 bell peppers, halved and seeds removed
- 1 cup corn kernels
- 1 cup diced tomatoes
- 1/2 cup diced red onion
- 1 teaspoon cumin
- 1/2 teaspoon chili powder
- Salt and black pepper to taste
- Fresh cilantro for garnish

Instructions:

1. Preheat the oven to 375°F (190°C).
2. In a bowl, mix cooked quinoa, black beans, corn kernels, diced tomatoes, diced red onion, cumin, chili powder, salt, and black pepper.
3. Stuff bell pepper halves with the quinoa and black bean mixture.
4. Bake for about 25-30 minutes or until peppers are tender.
5. Garnish with fresh cilantro before serving.

Nutritional Information (per serving): 400kcal; Fat: 5g; Carbs: 75g; Protein: 15g

Lentil and Vegetable Curry

Preparation time: 20 minutes

Cooking time: 40 minutes

Servings: 2

Ingredients:

- 1 cup dry lentils, rinsed and drained
- 2 cups mixed vegetables (carrots, peas, bell peppers)
- 1 onion, chopped
- 2 cloves garlic, minced
- 1 can (14 oz) diced tomatoes
- 1 can (14 oz) coconut milk
- 2 tablespoons curry powder
- 1 teaspoon turmeric
- Salt and black pepper to taste
- Fresh cilantro for garnish

Instructions

1. In a pot, combine lentils, mixed vegetables, chopped onion, minced garlic, diced tomatoes, coconut milk, curry powder, turmeric, salt, and black pepper.
2. Bring to a boil, then reduce heat and simmer for about 30-40 minutes.
3. Serve over rice or quinoa.
4. Garnish with fresh cilantro before serving.

Nutritional Information (per serving): 450kcal; Fat: 15g; Carbs: 60g; Protein: 20g

Zucchini Noodles with Vegan Pesto

Preparation time: 15 minutes

Cooking time: 10 minutes

Servings: 2

Ingredients:

- 2 large zucchinis, spiralized into noodles
- 1 cup cherry tomatoes, halved
- 1/2 cup pine nuts
- 2 cups fresh basil leaves
- 2 cloves garlic
- 1/2 cup nutritional yeast
- 1/2 cup olive oil
- Salt and black pepper to taste
- Lemon wedges for serving

Instructions:

1. In a blender or food processor, combine pine nuts, basil leaves, garlic, nutritional yeast, olive oil, salt, and black pepper. Blend until smooth.
2. In a pan, sauté zucchini noodles until just tender.
3. Toss zucchini noodles with vegan pesto and cherry tomatoes.
4. Serve with lemon wedges.

Nutritional Information (per serving): 350kcal; Fat: 30g; Carbs: 15g; Protein: 10g

Chickpea and Spinach Coconut Curry

Preparation time: 15 minutes

Cooking time: 25 minutes

Servings: 2

Ingredients:

- 1 can (14 oz) chickpeas, drained and rinsed
- 2 cups fresh spinach
- 1 onion, chopped
- 2 cloves garlic, minced
- 1 can (14 oz) diced tomatoes
- 1 can (14 oz) coconut milk
- 2 tablespoons curry powder
- 1 teaspoon cumin
- Salt and black pepper to taste
- Fresh cilantro for garnish

Instructions:

1. In a pan, sauté chopped onion and minced garlic until softened.
2. Add chickpeas, fresh spinach, diced tomatoes, coconut milk, curry powder, cumin, salt, and black pepper.
3. Simmer for about 20-25 minutes.
4. Serve over rice or quinoa.
5. Garnish with fresh cilantro before serving.

Nutritional Information (per serving): 400kcal; Fat: 20g; Carbs: 50g; Protein: 15g

Roasted Vegetable and Hummus Wrap

Preparation time: 15 minutes

Cooking time: 20 minutes

Servings: 2

Ingredients:

- 2 whole-grain wraps
- 1 cup mixed vegetables (bell peppers, zucchini, red onion), sliced
- 1 tablespoon olive oil
- Salt and black pepper to taste
- 1/2 cup hummus
- Fresh spinach leaves
- Cherry tomatoes, sliced
- Feta cheese (optional)

Instructions:

1. Preheat the oven to 400°F (200°C).
2. Toss mixed vegetables with olive oil, salt, and black pepper.
3. Roast in the oven for about 15-20 minutes or until vegetables are tender.
4. Spread hummus on each wrap.
5. Fill wraps with roasted vegetables, fresh spinach, cherry tomatoes, and optional feta cheese.
6. Roll up and enjoy!

Nutritional Information (per serving): 350kcal; Fat: 15g; Carbs: 45g; Protein: 10g

Sweet Potato and Black Bean Enchiladas

Preparation time: 25 minutes

Cooking time: 30 minutes

Servings: 2

Ingredients:

- 4 whole-grain tortillas
- 2 sweet potatoes, peeled and diced
- 1 can (14 oz) black beans, drained and rinsed
- 1 cup corn kernels
- 1 cup enchilada sauce
- 1 cup shredded cheddar cheese
- Fresh cilantro for garnish
- Greek yogurt for serving

Instructions:

1. Preheat the oven to 375°F (190°C).
2. Boil or steam sweet potatoes until tender.
3. In a bowl, mix sweet potatoes, black beans, and corn.
4. Fill tortillas with the mixture, roll, and place in a baking dish.
5. Pour enchilada sauce over the top and sprinkle with shredded cheddar cheese.
6. Bake for about 25-30 minutes or until cheese is melted and bubbly.
7. Garnish with fresh cilantro and serve with a dollop of Greek yogurt.

Nutritional Information (per serving): 400kcal; Fat: 10g; Carbs: 60g; Protein: 15g

Mediterranean Chickpea Salad

Preparation time: 15 minutes

Cooking time: 0 minutes

Servings: 2

Ingredients:

- 1 can (14 oz) chickpeas, drained and rinsed
- 1 cup cherry tomatoes, halved
- 1 cucumber, diced
- 1/2 red onion, finely chopped
- 1/2 cup Kalamata olives, sliced
- 1/2 cup crumbled feta cheese
- Fresh parsley, chopped
- 2 tablespoons olive oil
- 1 tablespoon red wine vinegar
- Salt and black pepper to taste

Instructions:

1. In a large bowl, combine chickpeas, cherry tomatoes, cucumber, red onion, olives, feta cheese, and parsley.
2. In a small bowl, whisk together olive oil, red wine vinegar, salt, and black pepper.
3. Drizzle the dressing over the salad and toss to combine.
4. Serve chilled.

Nutritional Information (per serving): 350kcal; Fat: 15g; Carbs: 40g; Protein: 15g

Portobello Mushroom and Quinoa Burgers

Preparation time: 20 minutes

Cooking time: 15 minutes

Servings: 2

Ingredients:

- 2 portobello mushroom caps
- 1 cup cooked quinoa
- 1/2 cup breadcrumbs
- 1/4 cup grated Parmesan cheese
- 2 cloves garlic, minced
- 1 teaspoon dried oregano
- Salt and black pepper to taste
- 2 whole-grain burger buns
- Lettuce, tomato slices, and condiments for topping

Instructions:

1. Preheat the grill or grill pan over medium heat.
2. In a bowl, combine cooked quinoa, breadcrumbs, Parmesan cheese, minced garlic, dried oregano, salt, and black pepper.
3. Remove the stems from portobello mushrooms and fill the caps with the quinoa mixture.
4. Grill for about 7-8 minutes per side or until mushrooms are tender.
5. Toast burger buns on the grill.
6. Assemble burgers with lettuce, tomato slices, and your favorite condiments.

Nutritional Information (per serving): 400kcal; Fat: 10g; Carbs: 60g; Protein: 20g

Vegan Thai Green Curry with Tofu

Preparation time: 15 minutes

Cooking time: 25 minutes

Servings: 2

Ingredients:

- 1 block (14 oz) extra-firm tofu, cubed
- 1 tablespoon coconut oil
- 1 onion, thinly sliced
- 2 bell peppers, sliced
- 1 zucchini, sliced
- 2 tablespoons green curry paste
- 1 can (14 oz) coconut milk
- 1 cup broccoli florets
- 1 cup snow peas
- 1 tablespoon soy sauce
- 1 tablespoon maple syrup
- Fresh cilantro for garnish
- Cooked jasmine rice for serving

Instructions:

1. Press tofu to remove excess water, then cube it.
2. In a large pan, heat coconut oil over medium heat and sauté tofu until golden brown.
3. Add sliced onion, bell peppers, and zucchini. Cook until vegetables are tender.
4. Stir in green curry paste and cook for 1-2 minutes.
5. Pour in coconut milk, add broccoli and snow peas, and simmer until vegetables are cooked.
6. Season with soy sauce and maple syrup. Adjust to taste.
7. Serve over cooked jasmine rice, garnished with fresh cilantro.

Nutritional Information (per serving: 450kcal; Fat: 30g; Carbs: 30g; Protein: 15g

Spinach and Mushroom Quinoa Risotto

Preparation time: 20 minutes

Cooking time: 25 minutes

Servings: 2

Ingredients:

- 1 cup quinoa, rinsed
- 2 cups vegetable broth
- 1 tablespoon olive oil
- 1 onion, finely chopped
- 2 cloves garlic, minced
- 8 oz mushrooms, sliced
- 4 cups fresh spinach
- 1/4 cup nutritional yeast
- Salt and black pepper to taste
- Lemon zest for garnish

Instructions:

1. In a saucepan, bring vegetable broth to a simmer.
2. In another pan, heat olive oil and sauté onion and garlic until softened.
3. Add mushrooms and cook until they release their moisture.
4. Stir in quinoa and cook for 1-2 minutes.
5. Begin adding the warm vegetable broth one ladle at a time, stirring frequently.
6. Continue adding broth until quinoa is cooked and creamy.
7. Fold in fresh spinach, nutritional yeast, salt, and black pepper.
8. Garnish with lemon zest before serving.

Nutritional Information (per serving): 400kcal; Fat: 10g; Carbs: 60g; Protein: 15g

Vegan Chickpea and Sweet Potato Chili

Preparation time: 15 minutes

Cooking time: 30 minutes

Servings: 2

Ingredients:

- 1 tablespoon olive oil
- 1 onion, chopped
- 2 cloves garlic, minced
- 1 sweet potato, diced
- 1 can (14 oz) chickpeas, drained and rinsed
- 1 can (14 oz) diced tomatoes
- 1 cup vegetable broth
- 1 tablespoon chili powder
- 1 teaspoon cumin
- 1/2 teaspoon smoked paprika
- Salt and black pepper to taste
- Avocado, cilantro, and lime for topping

Instructions:

1. In a large pot, heat olive oil and sauté onion and garlic until softened.
2. Add sweet potato, chickpeas, diced tomatoes, and vegetable broth.
3. Season with chili powder, cumin, smoked paprika, salt, and black pepper.
4. Bring to a boil, then reduce heat and simmer for 25-30 minutes.
5. Serve topped with sliced avocado, fresh cilantro, and a squeeze of lime.

Nutritional Information (per serving): 380kcal; Fat: 10g; Carbs: 60g; Protein: 12g

Chapter 9: Desserts

Dark Chocolate Avocado Mousse

Preparation time: 10 minutes

Cooking time: 0 minutes

Servings: 2

Ingredients:

- 2 ripe avocados
- 1/4 cup unsweetened cocoa powder
- 1/4 cup maple syrup
- 1 teaspoon vanilla extract
- A pinch of salt
- 1/4 cup almond milk
- Dark chocolate shavings for garnish

Instructions:

1. In a blender, combine avocados, cocoa powder, maple syrup, vanilla extract, salt, and almond milk.
2. Blend until smooth and creamy.
3. Divide the mousse into serving glasses.
4. Refrigerate for at least 2 hours.
5. Garnish with dark chocolate shavings before serving.

Nutritional Information (per serving): 250kcal; Fat: 16g; Carbs: 27g; Protein: 4g

Coconut Flour Banana Bread

Preparation time: 15 minutes

Cooking time: 45 minutes

Servings: 2

Ingredients:

- 2 ripe bananas, mashed
- 2 eggs
- 1/4 cup coconut oil, melted
- 1/4 cup coconut flour
- 1/2 teaspoon baking soda
- 1/2 teaspoon cinnamon
- A pinch of salt
- 1/4 cup chopped walnuts (optional)

Instructions:

1. Preheat the oven to 350°F (175°C) and grease a small loaf pan.
2. In a bowl, mix mashed bananas, eggs, and melted coconut oil.
3. Add coconut flour, baking soda, cinnamon, and salt. Stir until well combined.
4. Fold in chopped walnuts if using.
5. Pour the batter into the prepared loaf pan.
6. Bake for 40-45 minutes or until a toothpick comes out clean.
7. Allow to cool before slicing.

Nutritional Information (per serving): 320kcal; Fat: 20g; Carbs: 30g; Protein: 6g

Protein-Packed Peanut Butter Cookies

Preparation time: 10 minutes

Cooking time: 10 minutes

Servings: 2 dozen cookies

Ingredients:

- 1 cup peanut butter
- 1/2 cup protein powder (vanilla or chocolate)
- 1/2 cup honey
- 1 egg
- 1 teaspoon vanilla extract

Instructions:

1. Preheat the oven to 350°F (175°C) and line a baking sheet with parchment paper.
2. In a bowl, mix peanut butter, protein powder, honey, egg, and vanilla extract until well combined.
3. Scoop spoonfuls of dough and place them on the prepared baking sheet.
4. Flatten each cookie with a fork, creating a crisscross pattern.
5. Bake for 10 minutes or until the edges are golden.
6. Allow to cool before serving.

Nutritional Information (per cookie): 100kcal; Fat: 7g; Carbs: 8g; Protein: 4g

Lemon Blueberry Protein Muffins

Preparation time: 15 minutes

Cooking time: 20 minutes

Servings: 2 dozen muffins

Ingredients:

- 2 cups almond flour
- 1/2 cup protein powder (vanilla)
- 1 teaspoon baking powder
- 1/2 teaspoon baking soda
- A pinch of salt
- 1/4 cup coconut oil, melted
- 1/4 cup honey
- 1/2 cup unsweetened almond milk
- 2 eggs
- 1 teaspoon vanilla extract
- Zest of 1 lemon
- 1 cup fresh blueberries

Instructions:

1. Preheat the oven to 350°F (175°C) and line a muffin tin with paper liners.
2. In a large bowl, whisk together almond flour, protein powder, baking powder, baking soda, and salt.
3. In another bowl, mix melted coconut oil, honey, almond milk, eggs, vanilla extract, and lemon zest.
4. Combine the wet and dry ingredients, then fold in the blueberries.
5. Spoon the batter into the muffin tin, filling each cup about 2/3 full.
6. Bake for 18-20 minutes or until a toothpick comes out clean.
7. Allow to cool before serving.

Nutritional Information (per muffin): 100kcal; Fat: 8g; Carbs: 10g; Protein: 5g

Almond Flour Chocolate Chip Blondies

Preparation time: 15 minutes

Cooking time: 25 minutes

Servings: 2 dozen blondies

Ingredients:

- 2 cups almond flour
- 1/2 cup coconut sugar
- 1/2 teaspoon baking soda
- 1/4 teaspoon salt
- 1/2 cup melted coconut oil
- 2 eggs
- 1 teaspoon vanilla extract
- 1/2 cup chocolate chips

Instructions:

1. Preheat the oven to 350°F (175°C) and grease a baking pan.
2. In a bowl, combine almond flour, coconut sugar, baking soda, and salt.
3. In a separate bowl, whisk together melted coconut oil, eggs, and vanilla extract.
4. Mix the wet ingredients into the dry ingredients until well combined.
5. Fold in chocolate chips.
6. Spread the batter evenly in the prepared pan.
7. Bake for 20-25 minutes or until a toothpick comes out with a few moist crumbs.
8. Allow to cool before cutting into squares.

Nutritional Information (per blondie): 120kcal; Fat: 8g; Carbs: 10g; Protein: 3g

Pumpkin Spice Energy Bites

Preparation time: 10 minutes

Cooking time: 0 minutes

Servings: 2 dozen bites

Ingredients:

- 1 cup rolled oats
- 1/2 cup pumpkin puree
- 1/4 cup almond butter
- 1/4 cup honey
- 1 teaspoon pumpkin spice
- 1/2 cup shredded coconut (for rolling)

Instructions:

1. In a bowl, combine rolled oats, pumpkin puree, almond butter, honey, and pumpkin spice.
2. Mix until the ingredients form a sticky dough.
3. Scoop small portions and roll them into bite-sized balls.
4. Roll each ball in shredded coconut to coat.
5. Refrigerate for at least 30 minutes before serving.

Nutritional Information (per bite): 60kcal; Fat: 3g; Carbs: 8g; Protein: 2g

Apple Cinnamon Quinoa Bake

Preparation time: 20 minutes

Cooking time: 30 minutes

Servings: 2

Ingredients:

- 1 cup cooked quinoa
- 2 apples, peeled and diced
- 1 teaspoon cinnamon
- 1/4 cup maple syrup
- 1/4 cup almond milk
- 2 eggs
- 1 teaspoon vanilla extract

Instructions:

1. Preheat the oven to 350°F (175°C) and grease a baking dish.
2. In a bowl, combine cooked quinoa, diced apples, cinnamon, maple syrup, almond milk, eggs, and vanilla extract.
3. Mix well and pour into the prepared baking dish.
4. Bake for 25-30 minutes or until set and golden brown.
5. Allow to cool slightly before serving.

Nutritional Information (per serving): 220kcal; Fat: 6g; Carbs: 36g; Protein: 7g

Avocado Chocolate Pudding Cups

Preparation time: 10 minutes

Cooking time: 0 minutes

Servings: 2

Ingredients:

- 2 ripe avocados
- 1/4 cup unsweetened cocoa powder
- 1/4 cup maple syrup
- 1 teaspoon vanilla extract
- A pinch of salt
- Fresh berries for topping

Instructions:

1. In a blender, combine avocados, cocoa powder, maple syrup, vanilla extract, and salt.
2. Blend until smooth and creamy.
3. Divide the pudding into serving cups.
4. Refrigerate for at least 1 hour.
5. Top with fresh berries before serving.

Nutritional Information (per serving): 200kcal; Fat: 14g; Carbs: 20g; Protein: 3g

Vanilla Protein Ice Cream

Preparation time: 10 minutes

Cooking time: 0 minutes

Freezing time: 4 hours

Servings: 2

Ingredients:

- 2 frozen bananas, sliced
- 1 cup unsweetened almond milk
- 1 scoop vanilla protein powder
- 1 teaspoon vanilla extract
- Optional toppings: chopped nuts, berries

Instructions:

1. In a blender, combine frozen banana slices, almond milk, vanilla protein powder, and vanilla extract.
2. Blend until smooth and creamy.
3. Pour the mixture into a freezer-safe container and freeze for at least 4 hours or until firm.
4. Scoop and serve with your favorite toppings.

Nutritional Information (per serving): 150kcal; Fat: 3g; Carbs: 25g; Protein: 10g

Mango Coconut Rice Pudding

Preparation time: 10 minutes

Cooking time: 25 minutes

Servings: 2

Ingredients:

- 1/2 cup arborio rice
- 2 cups coconut milk
- 1/4 cup maple syrup
- 1 teaspoon vanilla extract
- 1 cup ripe mango, diced
- Shredded coconut for garnish

Instructions:

1. In a saucepan, combine arborio rice, coconut milk, maple syrup, and vanilla extract.
2. Bring to a simmer over medium heat, then reduce heat to low, cover, and simmer for 20-25 minutes or until the rice is tender.
3. Stir in diced mango.
4. Remove from heat and let it cool.
5. Refrigerate for at least 2 hours before serving.
6. Garnish with shredded coconut before serving.

Nutritional Information (per serving): 300kcal; Fat: 10g; Carbs: 50g; Protein: 3g

Chapter 10:
Dining Out and Social Events

Here is a list of tips when you decide to dine out:

1. Smart Choices at the Sushi Bar
2. Navigating Carb Cycling at Italian Restaurants
3. Healthy Grilling Options for BBQs
4. Carb-Friendly Mexican Cuisine
5. Plant-Based Picks at Your Favorite Eatery
6. Mediterranean Delights: A Carb Cycling Guide
7. Making Wise Choices at Asian Fusion Restaurants
8. Ordering Low-Carb at Fast Food Joints
9. Carb Cycling on the Go: Healthy Takeout Options
10. Salad Strategies for Dining Out
11. Carb-Conscious Choices at Family Gatherings
12. Savoring Low-Carb Indian Cuisine
13. Carb Cycling at Brunch: Tips and Tricks
14. Staying on Track at Social Events
15. Enjoying Dessert without Breaking the Cycle

Chapter 11:
Approach for Long-Term Success

Fostering a sustainable and effective approach for long-term success is paramount. This chapter serves as a comprehensive guide, steering you away from short-lived fad diets and towards a balanced and adaptable lifestyle. We understand that the journey to optimal health and fitness is not a sprint but a marathon, and our goal is to equip you with the tools for lasting success.

One key aspect of the approach for long-term success is recognizing that carb cycling is not a one-size-fits-all solution. Individualization is at the core of sustained progress. This chapter delves into the importance of understanding your body's unique responses, preferences, and requirements. It provides practical strategies for adjusting your carb cycling plan over time, ensuring that it evolves with your changing needs and goals.

Moreover, we explore the significance of lifestyle integration. Carb cycling isn't just about what you eat; it's about how you live. We offer insights into seamlessly incorporating carb cycling into your daily routine, from grocery shopping and meal preparation to dining out and navigating social events. This holistic approach ensures that carb cycling becomes a natural and enjoyable part of your lifestyle, contributing to its long-term sustainability.

As we guide you through troubleshooting and overcoming plateaus, we emphasize the importance of patience and persistence. Plateaus are a normal part of any fitness journey, and this chapter equips you with strategies to navigate and overcome these challenges. By setting realistic expectations and celebrating small victories, you'll stay motivated on the path to long-term success.

In conclusion, the approach for long-term success in carb cycling goes beyond the immediate goals. It's about cultivating a mindset and lifestyle that support your well-being for years to come. This chapter empowers you with the knowledge and strategies needed to make carb cycling a sustainable and fulfilling part of your health and fitness journey.

2. Bonus Chapters:

1. Creating Balanced and Nutrient-Dense Meals

A pivotal aspect guiding sustained success is the creation of balanced and nutrient-dense meals. The philosophy behind this approach revolves around meticulously combining macronutrients—proteins, carbohydrates, and fats—in a way that not only supports your fitness goals but also prioritizes overall health and well-being.

Balanced meals play a crucial role in optimizing energy levels and enhancing metabolic efficiency. The careful distribution of macronutrients ensures a steady release of energy throughout the day, preventing energy crashes and promoting sustained vitality. This is particularly significant in the Carb Cycling framework, where the cyclical variation of carbohydrate intake is strategically employed to harness the benefits of both high and low carb days.

Nutrient density, on the other hand, focuses on maximizing the nutritional value per calorie consumed. The goal is to incorporate a variety of nutrient-rich foods, such as lean proteins, whole grains, colorful vegetables, and healthy fats, into your meals. These foods provide a spectrum of essential vitamins, minerals, antioxidants, and fiber that support various bodily functions, enhance recovery, and contribute to long-term health.

Creating balanced and nutrient-dense meals involves thoughtful meal planning and preparation. Begin by understanding your daily energy requirements, considering factors like activity level, fitness goals, and individual metabolism. Tailor your meals to align with the specific demands of high and low carb days, ensuring that your nutritional intake complements the cyclical nature of Carb Cycling.

Embracing a diverse range of food sources adds both flavor and nutritional depth to your meals. Experiment with colorful vegetables, lean proteins, whole grains, and healthy fats to craft meals that are not only satisfying but also promote optimal nutrition. The inclusion of a variety of foods ensures that you receive a broad spectrum of essential nutrients, fostering a holistic approach to health.

In essence, the art of creating balanced and nutrient-dense meals within the Carb Cycling Diet is a personalized journey. It empowers you to cultivate a positive relationship with food, fueling your body with the nutrients it needs to thrive. As you embark on this culinary adventure, remember that the key lies in thoughtful choices, variety, and a commitment to nourishing your body for sustained well-being.

Balanced and Nutrient-Dense Meal Examples

High Carb Day:

Example 1

Meal	Components
Breakfast	Quinoa Porridge with Berries and Almond Butter
Snack	Greek Yogurt Parfait with Granola and Mixed Nuts
Lunch	Sweet Potato and Chickpea Buddha Bowl with Avocado
Snack	Fresh Fruit Smoothie with Protein Powder
Dinner	Whole Wheat Pasta Primavera with Grilled Chicken

Example 2

Meal	Components
Breakfast	Oatmeal with Sliced Banana and Chia Seeds
Snack	Whole Grain Toast with Peanut Butter and Banana Slices
Lunch	Quinoa Salad with Roasted Vegetables and Feta Cheese
Snack	Mango and Pineapple Smoothie with Greek Yogurt and Flaxseeds
Dinner	Brown Rice Bowl with Black Beans, Corn, Avocado, and Grilled Chicken

Example 3

Meal	Components
Breakfast	Pancakes made with Whole Wheat Flour and Blueberries
Snack	Apple Slices with Almond Butter and Pumpkin Seeds
Lunch	Spaghetti with Tomato Sauce, Lean Ground Turkey, and Whole Wheat Pasta
Snack	Mixed Berry Parfait with Cottage Cheese and Granola
Dinner	Quinoa-Stuffed Bell Peppers with Lean Ground Beef and Tomato Sauce

Low Carb Day:

Example 1

Meal	Components
Breakfast	Scrambled Eggs with Spinach and Feta Cheese
Snack	Cottage Cheese with Cherry Tomatoes and Basil
Lunch	Grilled Salmon Salad with Mixed Greens and Olive Oil Dressing
Snack	Raw Veggies with Hummus
Dinner	Cauliflower Rice Stir-Fry with Tofu and Vegetables

Example 2

Meal	Components
Breakfast	Scrambled Eggs with Spinach and Feta Cheese
Snack	Celery Sticks with Creamy Hummus
Lunch	Grilled Salmon Salad with Mixed Greens and Avocado
Snack	Cucumber Slices with Tzatziki Dip
Dinner	Zucchini Noodles with Pesto and Grilled Shrimp

Example 3

Meal	Components
Breakfast	Keto-Friendly Smoothie with Coconut Milk, Berries, and Protein Powder
Snack	Hard-Boiled Eggs with a Side of Almonds
Lunch	Chicken Caesar Salad with Romaine Lettuce and Parmesan Cheese
Snack	Greek Yogurt with Chia Seeds and Sliced Strawberries
Dinner	Cauliflower Rice Stir-Fry with Tofu and Vegetables

These meal examples showcase the strategic combination of macronutrients (carbohydrates, proteins, and fats) to align with the high or low carb focus of the day. The high carb day includes complex carbohydrates to replenish glycogen stores, while the low carb day emphasizes protein and healthy fats for sustained energy.

Tips for Creating Balanced and Nutrient-Dense Meals:

1. Incorporate Lean Proteins: Include sources like poultry, fish, tofu, and legumes to support muscle maintenance.
2. Colorful Vegetables: Opt for a variety of colorful vegetables to ensure a broad spectrum of vitamins and minerals.
3. Healthy Fats: Include sources like avocados, nuts, seeds, and olive oil for satiety and overall health.
4. Whole Grains: Choose whole grains like quinoa, brown rice, and whole wheat for high carb days.
5. Hydration: Drink plenty of water and consider herbal teas to stay hydrated without added sugars.

Remember, these are general examples, and individual nutritional needs may vary. Adjust portions and specific food choices based on personal preferences, dietary restrictions, and fitness goals.

2. Advanced Strategies: Graduating to Advanced Carb Cycling

As you progress on your carb cycling journey, the chapter on "Advanced Strategies: Graduating to Advanced Carb Cycling" serves as your gateway to a new level of precision and optimization. This advanced phase is not just about adhering to a diet but rather mastering the art of carb cycling to achieve exceptional results tailored to your individual needs.

Understanding Individualization:

In this chapter, we delve into the importance of individualization in advanced carb cycling. Recognizing that each body responds uniquely to nutritional strategies, we explore how to fine-tune your approach based on factors such as metabolism, activity level, and specific fitness objectives.

Optimizing Carbohydrate Timing:

One key focus is on optimizing the timing of carbohydrate intake. The chapter provides insights into strategically adjusting your carb cycles to align with your daily activities and energy needs. By incorporating illustrative tables, you can visualize how timing adjustments can enhance fat utilization, support muscle development, and improve overall performance.

Fine-Tuning for Specific Goals:

Tailoring your approach becomes paramount in the advanced phase. Whether your goal is fat loss, muscle gain, or athletic performance, this chapter guides you on how to customize your carb cycling plan accordingly. The included tables offer practical examples, showcasing how adjustments in carbohydrate quantity and type can be made to cater to diverse fitness objectives.

Advanced Monitoring and Adjustment:

Achieving mastery in carb cycling requires a keen understanding of your body's responses. The chapter provides a detailed exploration of advanced monitoring techniques, empowering you to assess your progress and make informed adjustments. The accompanying tables provide a visual representation of how to tweak your carb cycling plan based on ongoing results.

Integration with Workout Routine:

To elevate your fitness routine, the chapter offers insights on seamlessly integrating advanced carb cycling with your workouts. Specific meal plans are provided for various fitness goals, demonstrating how your nutrition strategy can complement and enhance your exercise regimen.

Through individualization, optimized timing, and advanced customization, you'll gain the knowledge and tools needed to shape your nutrition plan with precision. The illustrative tables serve as practical aids, making the advanced strategies accessible and applicable to your unique fitness journey. Elevate your carb cycling experience and embark on a path to unparalleled health and fitness.

Conclusion

In conclusion "The New Carb Cycling for Beginners" isn't just a guide—it's your gateway to transformative health and fitness. As you turn the final pages of this comprehensive resource, you've not only gained an understanding of the fundamental principles of carb cycling but also acquired the tools to implement this dynamic dietary approach seamlessly into your life.

Embarking on this journey, you've unraveled the mysteries behind controlled carbohydrate consumption. The book has provided you with a roadmap, expertly crafted for beginners, guiding you through the intricacies of carb cycling with clarity and precision. Authored by seasoned professionals in the field, the content demystifies the science and empowers you to take control of your body composition and overall well-being.

Diving into the science behind carb cycling, you've unlocked the secrets to optimizing your energy levels, accelerating fat loss, and building lean muscle. The transformative power of this approach has been laid bare, offering you the opportunity to reshape your approach to nutrition and fitness.

Practical insights, customizable meal plans, and workout strategies have been presented to make carb cycling an integral part of your lifestyle. Whether you started as a fitness novice or someone looking to break through a plateau, the book has provided actionable tips to help you achieve your health and fitness goals.

Going beyond traditional dieting norms, "The New Carb Cycling for Beginners" advocates for sustainable and enjoyable nutrition practices. Clear explanations and practical guidance empower you to create balanced and nutrient-dense meals, making carb cycling an organic and fulfilling aspect of your daily life.

The journey doesn't end here; it extends into troubleshooting, overcoming plateaus, and adjusting your approach for long-term success. Common challenges have been addressed, solutions provided, and a roadmap for lifestyle integration has been laid out, ensuring that carb cycling seamlessly becomes part of your daily routine.

As you approach the conclusion of this transformative resource, consider this not the end but the beginning of a new chapter in your health and fitness journey

Manufactured by Amazon.ca
Acheson, AB